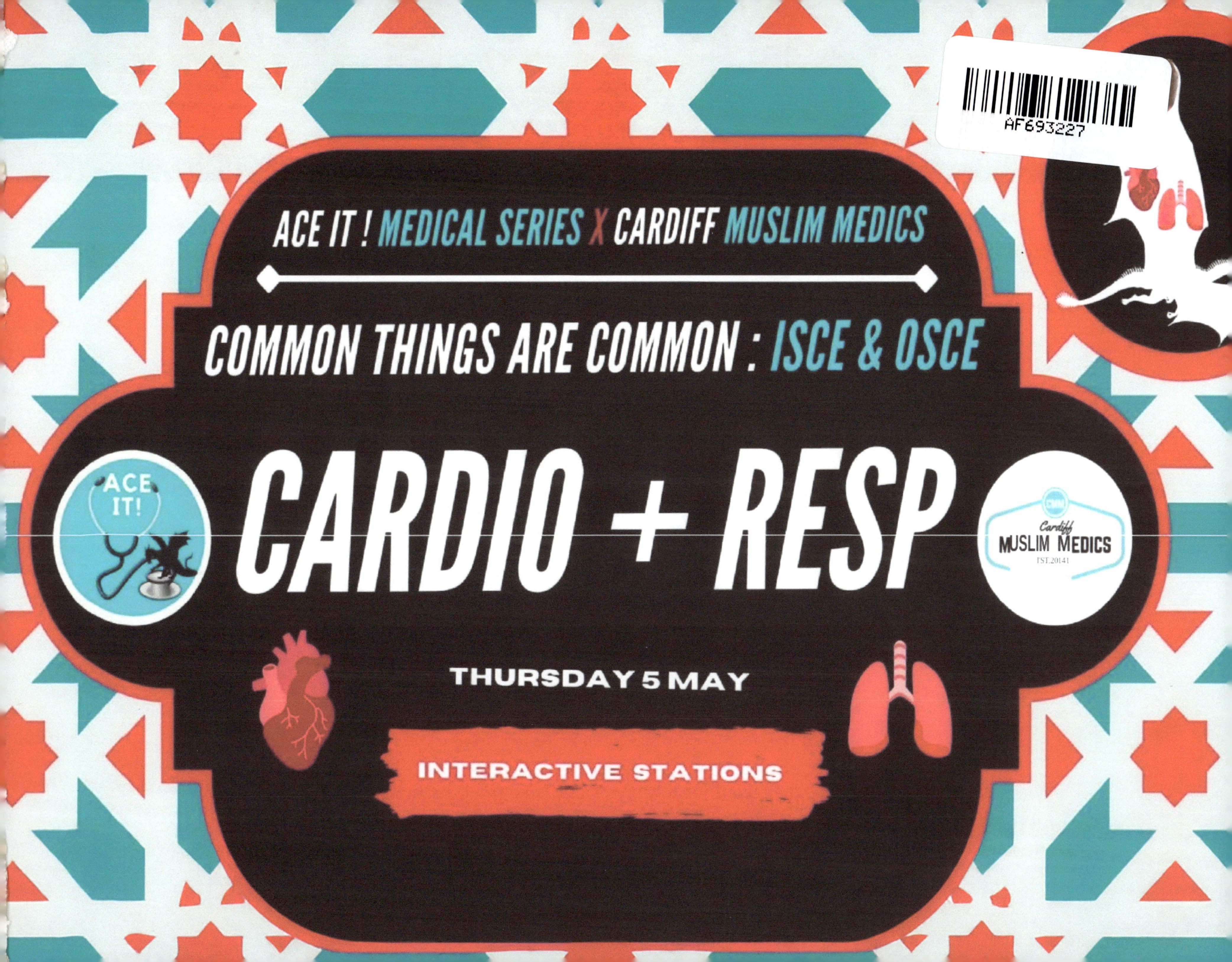
ACE IT ! MEDICAL SERIES X CARDIFF MUSLIM MEDICS
COMMON THINGS ARE COMMON : ISCE & OSCE
ACE IT!
CARDIO + RESP
Cardiff MUSLIM MEDICS
THURSDAY 5 MAY
INTERACTIVE STATIONS

OSCE Handbook – Ace it! Medical Series PART 2

Authors: Danyal Ahmed, Huria Metezai, Saif Abbas Chatoo, Abdullah ElBedawy, Abeer Zahid, Ahmed Fadil Bilal

First Published in 2026

ISBN: 978-1-80723-208-5 (Paperback)
978-1-80723-207-8 (E-Book)

Book cover design and Book layout by:
White Magic Studios
www.whitemagicstudios.co.uk

Published by:
Maple Publishers
Fairbourne Drive, Atterbury,
Milton Keynes,
MK10 9RG, UK
www.maplepublishers.com

A CIP catalogue record for this title is available from the British Library.

Table of Content

Station 5 – Explaining SSRIs

You are a medical student in a GP clinic. Mrs. L is a 45-year-old patient who has recently been diagnosed with moderate depression. Following a discussion with the GP, she has been prescribed a selective serotonin reuptake inhibitor (SSRI) and would like to understand more about the medication.

Your task: Please explain what SSRIs are, how they work, and what Mrs. L can expect from the treatment. You should discuss potential benefits, common side effects, how long they take to work, and address any concerns she may have. Check her understanding and offer reassurance where appropriate.

The examiner will stop you at 7 minutes, ask you a few questions, and ask you to summarise the consultation.

Mock OSCE Script: Explaining SSRIs to a Patient

Station Title: You are a medical student in a GP clinic. A patient has just been prescribed an SSRI for depression and wants to understand more about the medication. Please explain the treatment and address any concerns they may have.

🧑‍⚕️ **Candidate:**

Hello, my name is [Candidate Name], I'm one of the medical students working with the team today. I understand you've been prescribed a medication called an SSRI for your mood. Would it be okay if I explain what that is and how it works?

🧑🤝🧑 **Patient:**

Yes please. I don't really know much about it.

◈ **ACTION – How the Drug Works**

Candidate: No problem. SSRIs—short for selective serotonin reuptake inhibitors—are a type of antidepressant. They work by increasing the levels of a chemical called serotonin in your brain. Serotonin helps regulate mood, and by boosting it, SSRIs can help improve symptoms of depression and anxiety.

Does that make sense so far?

◈ **TIMING – When to Take It**

Candidate: You'll usually take the tablet once a day. Some people take it in the morning, others prefer the evening—your doctor will advise what's best for you.

◈ **HOW TO TAKE**

Candidate: You can take it with or without food, but try to take it at the same time each day to help build a routine.

◈ **LENGTH OF TREATMENT**

Candidate: It's important to know that this isn't a quick fix. It can take up to 4 weeks before you start noticing any improvement. Even then, the changes might be subtle at first—like having short periods of feeling a bit better.

Once you're feeling better, you'll usually continue the medication for at least 6 months to help prevent symptoms from coming back.

◈ EFFECTS – When It Starts Working

Candidate: As I mentioned, it can take a few weeks to start working. During that time, it's really important to keep taking it regularly, even if you're not feeling better straight away.

◈ TESTS – Monitoring

Candidate: We don't usually need blood tests for SSRIs, but your doctor will want to check in with you regularly—especially in the first few weeks—to see how you're getting on and to monitor for any side effects.

◈ SIDE EFFECTS

Candidate: Like all medications, SSRIs can cause side effects. Common ones include:

- Feeling sick or having an upset stomach
- Dry mouth
- Trouble sleeping
- Sweating
- Changes in sex drive
- Feeling your heart race or flutter

These often settle down after a few weeks. If they become difficult to cope with, let your doctor know—there are other options we can try.

◈ COMPLICATIONS & CONTRAINDICATIONS

Candidate: There are a few situations where SSRIs might not be suitable—for example, if someone has epilepsy, certain heart rhythm problems, or liver issues. Your doctor will have checked these before prescribing.

Also, SSRIs can interact with other medications—especially herbal remedies like St John's Wort—so it's important to let your doctor know about anything else you're taking.

◈ SUPPLEMENTARY ADVICE – Withdrawal & Safety-Netting

Candidate: SSRIs aren't addictive, but if you stop them suddenly, you might get withdrawal symptoms like restlessness, anxiety, or headaches. So if you ever want to stop, speak to your doctor first—they'll help you reduce the dose gradually.

One important thing to mention: sometimes, especially early on, people can feel more anxious or even have thoughts of hopelessness or self-harm. If that happens, it's really important to seek help straight away—either by calling your GP, NHS 111, or going to A&E if needed.

We'll also arrange a follow-up appointment—usually in 2–4 weeks, or sooner if needed—to check how you're doing.

❓ CHECKING UNDERSTANDING

Candidate: That was quite a bit of information—how are you feeling about it so far? Is there anything you'd like me to go over again?

Patient:

No, that was really helpful. Thank you.

Candidate (Closing):

You're very welcome. I'll make sure you get a leaflet with all this information, and we'll book that follow-up to see how you're getting on. If anything worries you in the meantime, please don't hesitate to reach out.

✅ Examiner Checklist Highlights

- Introduced self and confirmed patient's understanding
- Used ATHLETICS structure to explain treatment
- Delivered information in clear, non-medical language
- Used "chunk and check" technique throughout
- Explained mechanism, timing, duration, and effects
- Covered side effects, contraindications, and interactions
- Gave clear safety-netting advice
- Offered written information and follow-up
- Empathetic and patient-centred communication

❓ **CHECKING UNDERSTANDING**

Candidate: That was quite a bit of information—how are you feeling about it so far? Is there anything you'd like me to go over again?

🧑🤝🧑 **Patient:**

No, that was really helpful. Thank you.

🧑⚕️ **Candidate (Closing):**

You're very welcome. I'll make sure you get a leaflet with all this information, and we'll book that follow-up to see how you're getting on. If anything worries you in the meantime, please don't hesitate to reach out.

✅ **Examiner Checklist Highlights**

- Introduced self and confirmed patient's understanding
- Used ATHLETICS structure to explain treatment
- Delivered information in clear, non-medical language
- Used "chunk and check" technique throughout
- Explained mechanism, timing, duration, and effects
- Covered side effects, contraindications, and interactions
- Gave clear safety-netting advice
- Offered written information and follow-up
- Empathetic and patient-centred communication

Introduce yourself - Hello my name is and I am one of the medical students/Junior Doctors - working with the team today

Name the Drug and its Purpose:

Explain **why** the patient is being prescribed it.

"You've been prescribed *ramipril*, which is a medication used to lower blood pressure and protect your heart and kidneys."

How it works in simple terms - Avoid Jargon and use analogies if useful. For examples it realxes the

smooth muscles in the blood vessles making it easier for heart to pump blood

How to take it?

Include dose, frequency, route and timing.

You will take one tablet once a day ideally in the morning with water

Common and Serious Side effects: Mention 2–3 common ones and reassure.

"Some people experience a dry cough or dizziness, especially when starting the medication

Monitoring and Follow up: Mention any blood tests, BP checks, or reviews.

"We'll check your kidney function and potassium levels before and after starting the medication

Station 6 – Explaining a condition

OSCE: Rheumatoid Arthritis Diagnosis & Methotrexate Counselling

You are the FY1 doctor in the Rheumatology outpatient clinic. Ms. Alice Harris, a 54-year-old patient, has recently been diagnosed with rheumatoid arthritis following clinical assessment and blood tests. Your consultant has asked you to explain the diagnosis to her and counsel her on starting methotrexate as part of her treatment plan.

Your task: Please explain what rheumatoid arthritis is, including its nature as an autoimmune condition, typical symptoms, and long-term implications. Discuss the role of methotrexate in managing the disease, including how it works, how it's taken, potential side effects, and necessary monitoring. Address any concerns Ms. Harris may have and check her understanding throughout the consultation.

The examiner will stop you at 7 minutes, ask you a few questions, and ask you to summarise the consultation

👩‍⚕️ **Candidate:**

Hello Alice, I'm Dr [Candidate Name], one of the junior doctors working in the rheumatology team. I understand you've just seen the consultant and have been told you have rheumatoid arthritis. Would it be okay if I explain a bit more about what that means and talk through the treatment we're recommending?

Alice:

Yes, please. I'm still trying to take it all in.

◈ **Step 1: Explaining the Diagnosis**

Candidate: Of course. Rheumatoid arthritis is a condition where your immune system—normally there to protect you—starts attacking the lining of your joints by mistake. This causes inflammation, pain, stiffness, and sometimes swelling. Over time, if untreated, it can lead to joint damage.

It's different from osteoarthritis, which is more about wear and tear. Rheumatoid arthritis is an autoimmune condition, and it can affect people of any age.

Does that make sense so far?

◈ **Step 2: Introducing Methotrexate**

Candidate: To help manage this condition, we're recommending a medication called methotrexate. It's one of the most commonly used treatments for rheumatoid arthritis and works by calming down the immune system to reduce inflammation.

It's not a painkiller, but it helps prevent joint damage and flare-ups in the long term.

◈ **Step 3: How Methotrexate Is Taken**

Candidate: Methotrexate is usually taken once a week—either as a tablet or an injection. You'll also be given folic acid to take on a different day to help reduce side effects.

It's important to take it exactly as prescribed and not more often than once a week.

◈ **Step 4: How Long It Takes to Work**

Candidate: It can take about 6 to 12 weeks before you start noticing an improvement. So we'll monitor your symptoms and support you during that time.

◈ Step 5: Monitoring and Tests

Candidate: Because methotrexate affects your immune system and can impact your liver and blood cells, we'll need to do regular blood tests—usually every 2 to 4 weeks at first, then less often once things are stable.

This helps us make sure the medication is working safely.

◈ Step 6: Side Effects and Safety Advice

Candidate: Most people tolerate methotrexate well, but some common side effects include:

- Feeling sick
- Mouth ulcers
- Tiredness
- Increased risk of infections

Rarely, it can affect your liver or lungs, which is why we monitor you closely.

You'll need to avoid alcohol or keep it to a minimum, and you shouldn't take any over-the-counter medications—like ibuprofen—without checking with us first.

Also, methotrexate can harm a developing baby, so if there's any chance of pregnancy, we'll need to discuss contraception.

◈ Step 7: Supplementary Advice

Candidate: If you ever feel unwell—especially with signs of infection like fever or a persistent cough—please contact us or your GP straight away. We may need to pause the medication temporarily.

We'll also give you written information and arrange follow-up appointments to check how you're getting on.

Checking Understanding

Candidate: That was quite a bit of information—how are you feeling about it all? Is there anything you'd like me to go over again?

Alice:

It's a lot, but I think I understand. I'm just nervous about starting something new.

Candidate (Closing):

That's completely understandable, Alice. We'll be here to support you every step of the way. I'll make sure you get a leaflet with everything we've discussed, and we'll book your next appointment to check your bloods and see how you're doing.

Examiner Checklist Highlights

- Introduced self and confirmed patient's understanding
- Explained rheumatoid arthritis in simple terms
- Described methotrexate's role, dosing, and timeline
- Discussed monitoring and side effects clearly
- Provided safety-netting and supplementary advice
- Used "chunk and check" technique throughout
- Offered written information and follow-up

Introduction

1. Introduce yourself and confirm the patient's identity.
2. Check what the patient already knows or understands.
3. Ask permission to explain the condition.

Diagnosis

1. Clearly name the condition.
2. Use simple, non-medical language.
3. Avoid jargon unless the patient is familiar with it.

Cause

1. Briefly explain why the condition occurs.
2. Mention risk factors or underlying mechanisms if relevant.

Symptoms

1. Describe typical symptoms the patient may experience.
2. Relate them to the patient's own presentation if possible.

Investigations

1. Outline how the diagnosis was made (e.g., blood tests, imaging).
2. Mention any further tests needed to monitor or confirm.

Management

1. Explain treatment options: medical, surgical, lifestyle.
2. Discuss prognosis and expected outcomes.
3. Mention follow-up plans and support services.

Address Concerns

1. Invite questions or worries.
2. Respond empathetically and clarify misunderstandings.

Check Understanding

1. Ask the patient to summarise or reflect back key points.
2. Offer written information or resources if appropriate.

Safety Netting

1. Advise what to do if symptoms worsen or new ones develop.
2. Ensure the patient knows how to seek help

Station 5 – HRT counselling

You are the FY1 doctor in the outpatient clinic. Mrs. Amelia Wright is a 48-year-old woman attending to discuss hormone replacement therapy (HRT). She has had her last menstrual period over 18 months ago and is experiencing vasomotor symptoms, including hot flushes and night sweats.

Your task: Please explain what HRT is, including its role in managing menopausal symptoms. Discuss the benefits, risks, and different types of HRT available. Address any concerns Mrs. Wright may have, including long-term safety, and check her understanding throughout the consultation.

The examiner will stop you at 7 minutes, ask you a few questions, and ask you to summarise the consultation.

☐ Mock OSCE Script: HRT Counselling for Menopausal Symptoms

Station Title: You are an FY1 doctor in the outpatient clinic. Your next patient is Mrs Amelia Wright, a 48-year-old woman attending to discuss hormone replacement therapy (HRT). She has had her last menstrual period over 18 months ago and is experiencing vasomotor symptoms. Your task is to counsel her on HRT.

◈ Opening the Consultation

Candidate: Hello Mrs Wright, my name is Dr [Candidate Name], I'm one of the Foundation Year 1 doctors working in the clinic today. Could I just confirm your full name and date of birth?

Patient: Yes, Amelia Wright. 12th March 1977.

Candidate: Thank you. And is it okay if I call you Mrs Wright, or would you prefer something else?

Patient: Mrs Wright is fine.

Candidate: Great. I understand you're here today to talk about hormone replacement therapy. I'd like to ask you a few questions first, then explain what HRT is, how it works, and what the benefits and risks are. Is that okay with you?

Patient: Yes, that's fine.

◈ History Taking

Candidate: To start, could you tell me a bit about the symptoms you've been experiencing?

(Patient describes hot flushes, night sweats, trouble sleeping, and vaginal dryness.)

Candidate: Thank you for sharing that. Just to check, have you noticed any changes in your mood—such as feeling low, anxious, or irritable?

(Patient confirms mild mood changes.)

Candidate: Any changes in your sex drive or discomfort during intercourse?

(Patient mentions reduced libido and some discomfort.)

Candidate: Have you had any issues with memory or concentration?

(Patient says yes, occasionally.)

Candidate: Any urinary symptoms—like dryness, itching, needing to go more often, or infections?

(Patient confirms increased frequency and dryness.)

Candidate: And when was your last period?

Patient: About 18 months ago.

Candidate: Thank you. That would mean you're postmenopausal. Just a few more questions to make sure HRT is safe for you.

Do you have any history of breast, ovarian, or womb cancer?

(Patient says no.)

Any family history of breast cancer or heart disease?

(Patient says no.)

Are you taking any regular medications?

(Patient says no.)

Do you smoke or drink alcohol?

(Patient drinks occasionally, does not smoke.)

Do you stay physically active?

(Patient walks regularly.)

◈ Exploring Ideas, Concerns, and Expectations

Candidate: Can I ask—what do you already know about HRT?

(Patient says she's heard of it but doesn't know much.)

Candidate: Is there anything in particular that worries you about it?

(Patient is concerned about cancer risk.)

Candidate: And what are you hoping to get out of today's appointment? Are you looking for more information or hoping to start treatment?

(Patient says she's open to starting if it's safe.)

◈ Explaining HRT

Candidate: Thank you. HRT stands for hormone replacement therapy. Around menopause, your body's levels of oestrogen drop, which causes many of the symptoms you've described—like hot flushes, sleep problems, and vaginal dryness.

HRT works by replacing that oestrogen, helping to relieve those symptoms. It also has long-term benefits, like reducing your risk of heart disease and protecting your bones from osteoporosis.

For women who still have a womb, we also give a hormone called progestogen. This protects the lining of the womb from building up too much, which can happen if you take oestrogen alone.

◈ Types and Regimes

Candidate: There are different ways to take HRT. You can take it as a tablet (oral), or through the skin using patches or gels (transdermal). Patches and gels tend to have fewer risks, especially for blood clots.

Because you haven't had a period in over a year, we'd recommend a continuous combined regime. This means you take both hormones every day and shouldn't have any bleeding.

If you didn't have a womb, or had a Mirena coil, you could take oestrogen-only HRT.

◈ Benefits of HRT

Candidate: The main benefit is improving your symptoms—like the night sweats and vaginal dryness you mentioned. It also helps with mood, concentration, and libido.

◈ Risks of HRT

Candidate: There are **some** risks to be aware of. Oral HRT slightly increases the risk of blood clots and stroke, though the overall risk is still low. There's also a small increase in breast cancer risk with combined HRT, which is linked to the progestogen component.

If someone takes oestrogen-only HRT and still has a womb, there's a risk of womb cancer—so we always give progestogen alongside it.

◈ Side Effects

Candidate: Some women experience side effects, especially early on. These can include:

- Breast tenderness
- Nausea
- Headaches
- Mood swings
- Bloating
- Irregular bleeding

These often settle with time, and we can adjust the dose or type if needed.

◈ Alternatives to HRT

Candidate: There are alternatives if you decide not to start HRT. For hot flushes, we can use medications like SSRIs or clonidine. For vaginal dryness, lubricants and moisturisers can help. For mood symptoms, talking therapies or antidepressants may be useful.

◈ Contraindications Check

Candidate: Just to confirm, you don't have any history of breast cancer, womb cancer, blood clots, heart disease, or liver problems?

(Patient confirms no.)

◈ Checking Understanding and Closing

Candidate: Does that all make sense so far? Is there anything you'd like me to go over again?

(Patient says she understands and has no further questions.)

Candidate: Great. So today we spoke about hormone replacement therapy—what it is, how it's taken, the benefits, risks, and side effects. You've had your last period over 18 months ago and are experiencing menopausal symptoms. You have no contraindications to HRT, and you're open to starting treatment.

We'll give you some written information and arrange a follow-up to see how you're getting on. If you have any concerns, please don't hesitate to get in touch.

Introduction

Wash hands, don PPE if needed.
Introduce yourself with name and role.
Confirm patient identity (name and DOB).
Explain the purpose of the consultation.

Explore ICE

Ask what the patient knows: “Have you heard of HRT?”
Explore concerns: “Is there anything that worries you about HRT?”
Clarify expectations: “What were you hoping HRT might do for you?”

Explain HRT clearly

HRT is a treatment used to relieve menopause symptoms by replacing hormones like oestrogen and progesterone.”
“It can help with hot flushes, mood changes, and reduce long-term risks like osteoporosis.”

Discuss HRT types

Oral tablets
Skin patches
Gels
Implants (e.g., Mirena coil)
Vaginal oestrogen (for urogenital symptoms)

Benefits

Symptom relief (hot flushes, vaginal dryness, mood swings)
Reduced risk of osteoporosis and cardiovascular disease

Risks

VTE risk (higher with oral HRT, lower with transdermal)
Breast cancer risk (especially with combined HRT)
Side effects: bloating, breast tenderness, headaches

Tailoring treatment

Consider patient's age, medical history, uterus status (need for progestogen if uterus intact)
Discuss lifestyle advice: smoking, alcohol, exercise
Offer non-hormonal options if appropriate

Check Understanding & Summarize

- Ask if they have questions
- Recap key points
- Offer written information or follow-up

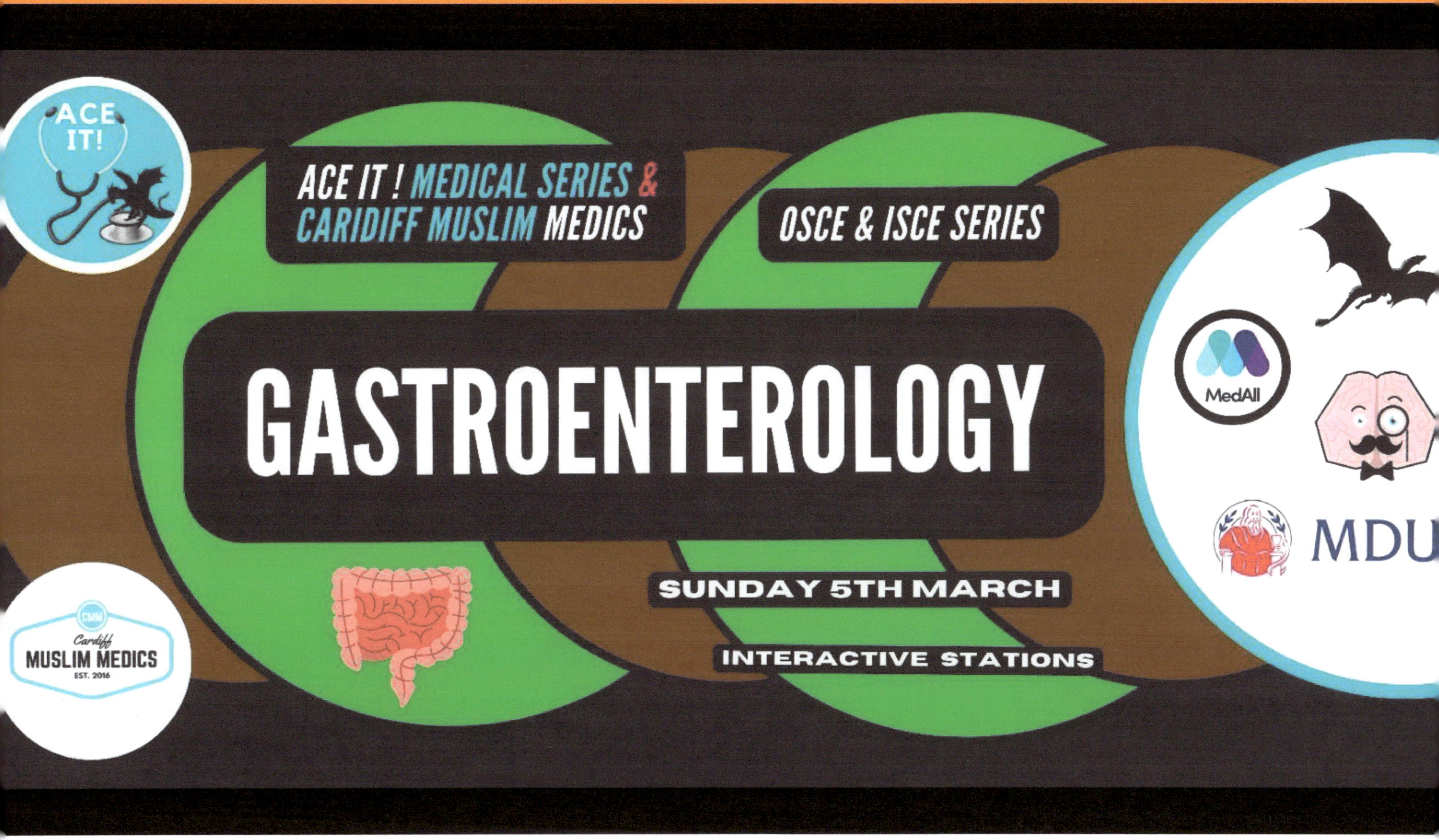
ACE IT!
ACE IT ! MEDICAL SERIES &
CARIDIFF MUSLIM MEDICS
OSCE & ISCE SERIES
GASTROENTEROLOGY
SUNDAY 5TH MARCH
INTERACTIVE STATIONS
MedAll
MDU
Cardiff
MUSLIM MEDICS
EST. 2016

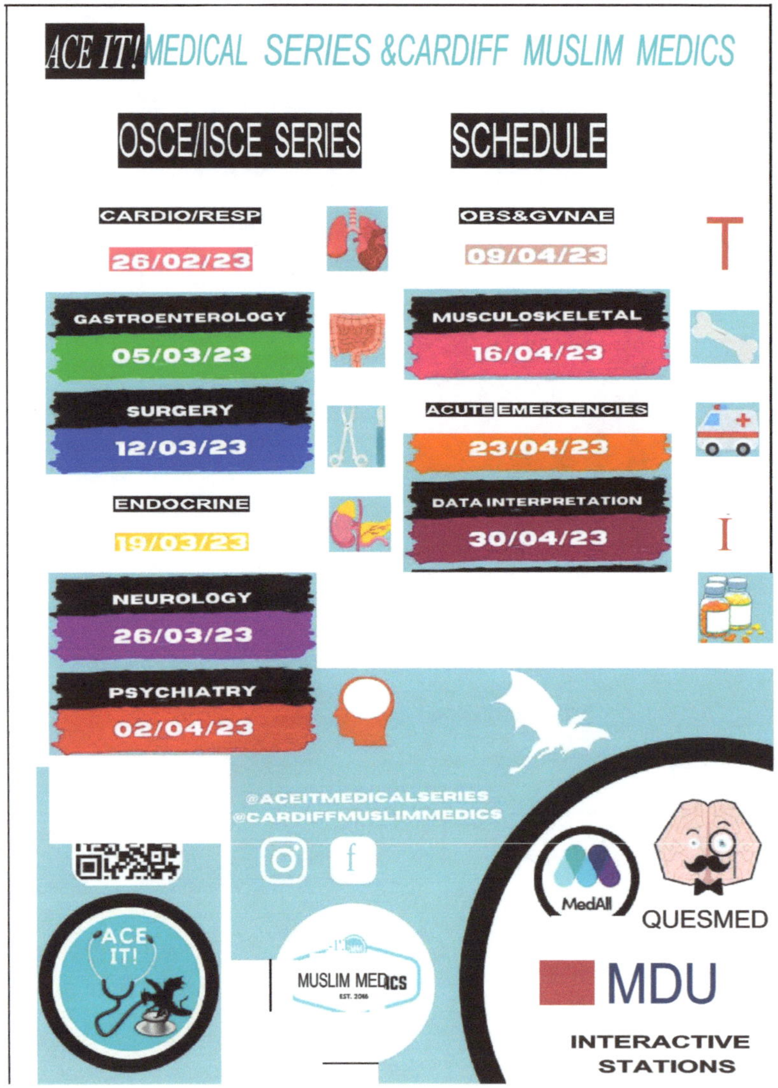
ACE IT! MEDICAL SERIES & CARDIFF MUSLIM MEDICS
OSCE/ISCE SERIES
SCHEDULE
CARDIO/RESP
26/02/23
OBS&GYNAE
09/04/23
GASTROENTEROLOGY
05/03/23
MUSCULOSKELETAL
16/04/23
SURGERY
12/03/23
ACUTE EMERGENCIES
23/04/23
ENDOCRINE
19/03/23
DATA INTERPRETATION
30/04/23
NEUROLOGY
26/03/23
PSYCHIATRY
02/04/23
@ACEITMEDICALSERIES
@CARDIFFMUSLIMMEDICS
ACE IT!
MUSLIM MEDICS
EST. 2016
MedAll
QUESMED
MDU
INTERACTIVE STATIONS

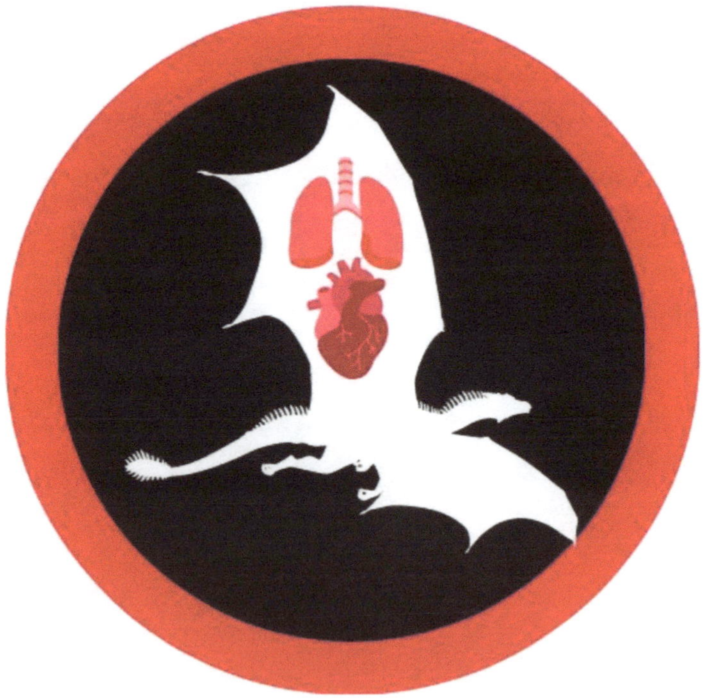

Learning Outcomes

To practice taking GI histories

To develop a framework for summaries and ongoing management plans

To revise some common GI conditions
(hidden for the sake of the cases)

Symptom explosions GI History

1) ABDOMINAL PAIN

SOCRATES
Site=organ

Travel/diet history

2) CHANGE IN BOWEL HABITS

Consistency
Colour
Course

If blood, how much and ?mixed with stools

Travel/diet history

3) VOMITING

Content- ?blood
Colour
Amount
Episodes

4) WEIGHT LOSS

How much?
Dress/clothes sizes, comments from others

How long? *>5% 6-12 months*

Intentional or unintentional

5) HAEMODYNAMIC COMPROMISE

Pale, light headed, dizzy, syncope, drowsy
Racing heart

Could indicate serious pathology

If female patient- take a brief obs and gynae overview (see next slide)

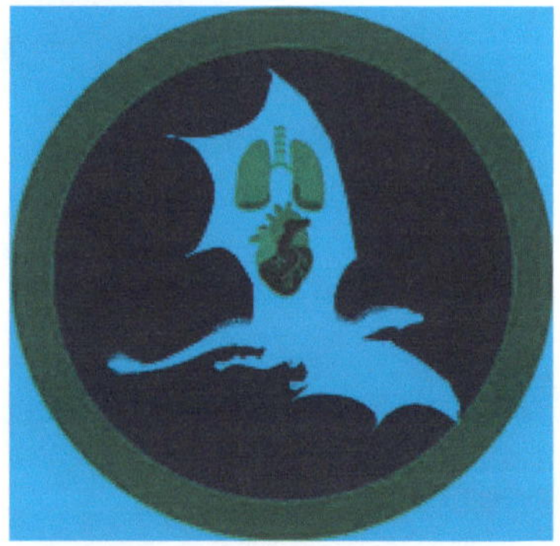

Upper GI paln History

1. PC
2. HoPC – **SOCRATES, change in bowel habits; if female, do a brief obs&gynae review**

   BSc MS: Births, Sexual history, Contraception, Menstruation, Smears

3. PMH/PSH- **Abdominal surgeries (=> adhesions)**
4. DHx – **Allergies!! Current medications and OTC (nb NSAIDs)**
5. FHx – **any GI conditions or cancers**
6. Social – **Travel/diet history, smoking, ALCOHOL, etc**
7. ICE
8. Systems review- **Top to toe**

In 4 min Hx for acute stations, key points are PC HPC + DHx should you run out of time

Some GI differentials to have in mind

1) STOMACH

Peptic ulcer disease
Gastroenteritis
Gastric cancer

2) OESOPHAGUS

GORD
- Oesophagitis
- Barret's

Oesophageal cancer
Pharyngeal pouch
Achalasia
Varices

3) PANCREAS

Acute pancreatitis
Chronic pancreatitis
Pancreatic cancer

4) BILIARY TREE

Biliary colic
Acute cholecystitis
Ascending cholangitis
Cholangiocarcinoma

5) SMALL INTESTINE (+Others)

Inferior MI
Abdominal Aortic Aneurysm
Acute mesenteric ischaemia
Ischaemic colitis

IBD (UC/Crohn's)
Coeliac's

Surgical Sieve

Question 1:Which system?
Question 2:Which organ?
Question 3:Which process?

Vitamin CDEF
Vascular
Inflammatory/infection
Trauma
Autoimmune
Metabolic
Iatrogenic
Neoplastic
Congenital
Drugs
Endocrine
Functional

Question 4:Why?

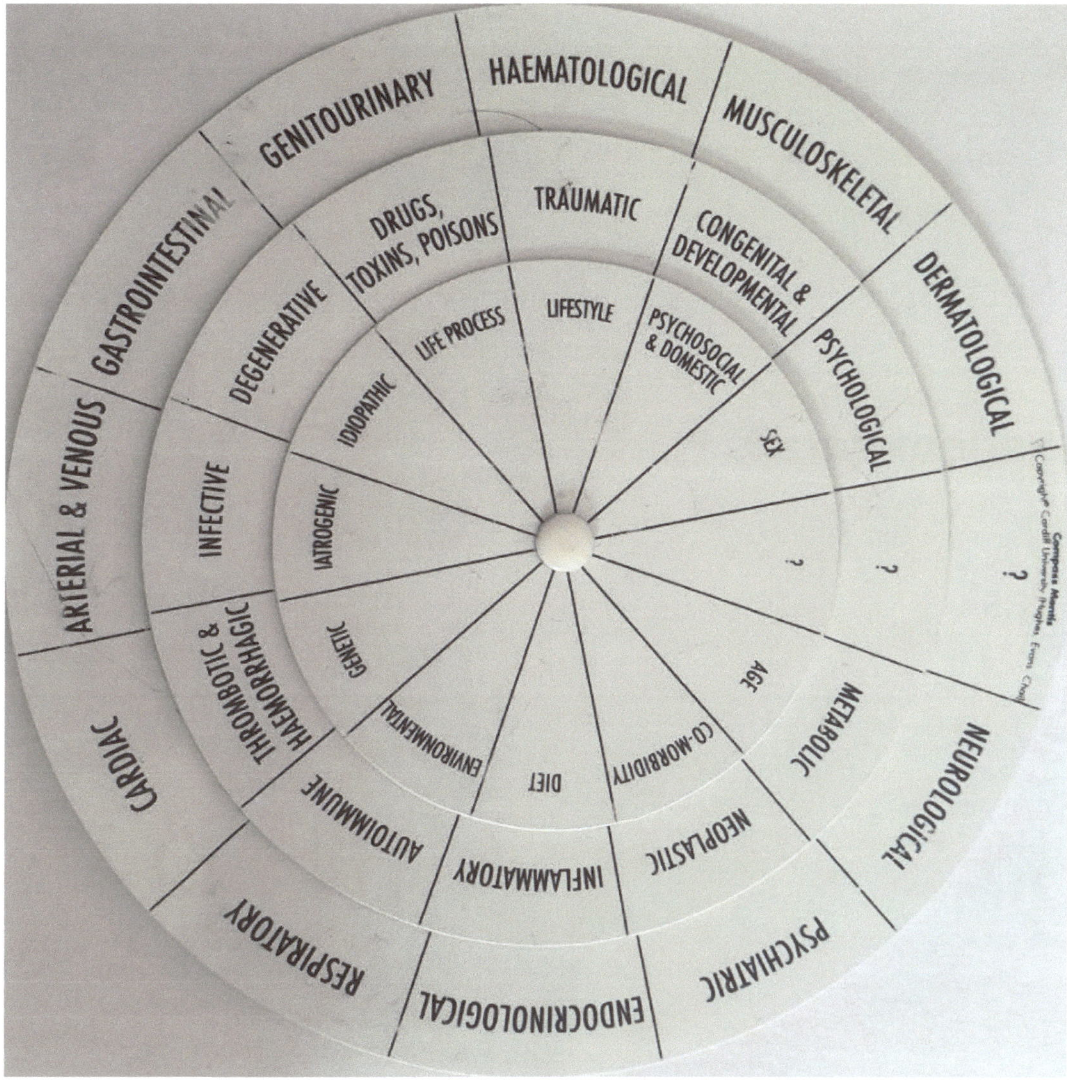

★ Station 1

Setting	**You are a 4th year medical student in the emergency department**
Patient details	**Yusuf a 52-year-old gentleman presents after vomiting fresh red blood.**
Task	**Please take a 4 min history**

Station 1

1) Please could you summarise your history and state your top 3 differentials.

Summary:

Patient name, age and presenting complaint

Follow history structure

Mention relevant positive findings Important negatives

Differentials

2) Which investigations would you request in this patient?

Differentials

Always give 3 – generally 2 of the most likely system involved and 1 of another

Looking at the patient demographic can give a clue but don't stereotype!

- **Acute Upper GI bleed**
- **Variceal bleed**
- **Peptic ulcer disease**
- **Mallory Weiss Tear**

Acute Upper GI bleed

Bleeding from the gastrointestinal tract proximal to the duodenum

Causes

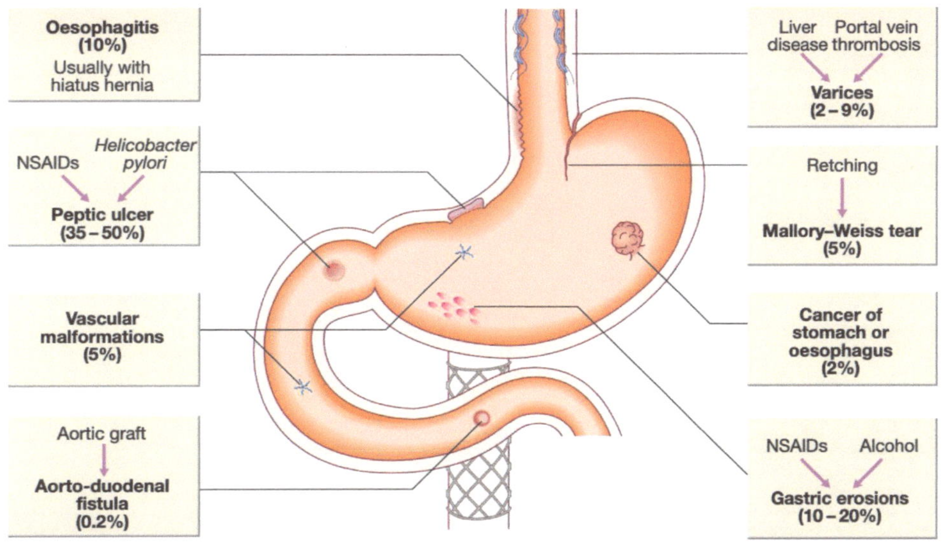

Fig. 21.19 Causes of acute upper gastrointestinal haemorrhage. Frequency is given in parentheses. (NSAIDs = non-steroidal anti-inflammatory drugs)

Symptoms

Haematemesis

Melaena

Symptoms of blood loss

Acute Upper GI bleed Ix

Key Investigations

Bedside-

Blatchford bleeding score

Used on admission to estimate need for intervention

Vital signs Bloods-

FBC, U&E, LFT,

Coagulation screen, crossmatch + G&S

Imaging- Endoscopy (w/i 24h, immediate if severe)

Framework for investigations:
BBOXES: Bedside, bloods, orifices, xrays, ?everything else, special tests Bedside, bloods, imaging, special tests

Acute Upper GI bleed Ix

Endoscopic image Name: X
DOB: 09-09-1971

Taken 05/03/2023

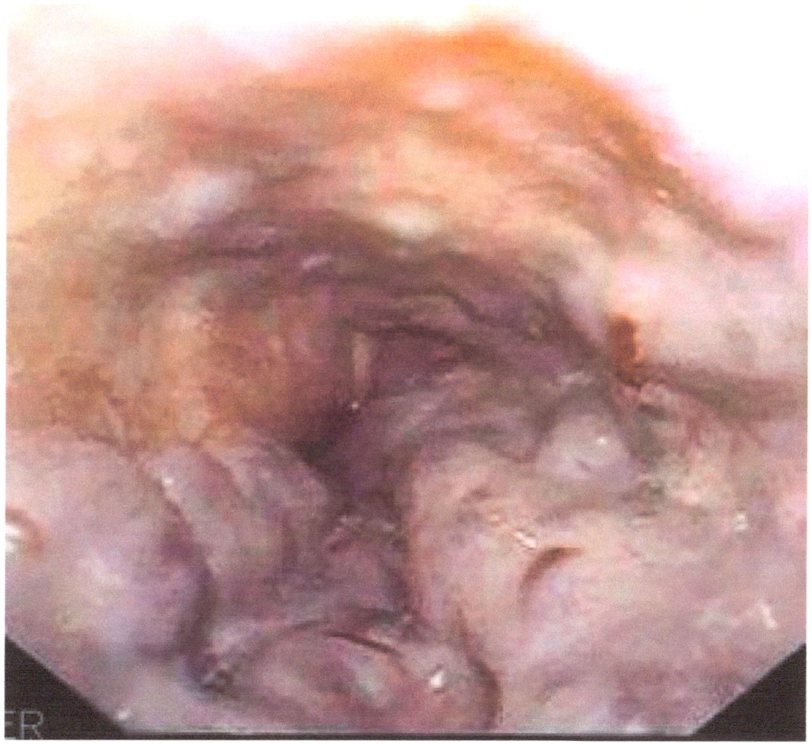

Please interpret the image above and formulate a management plan for the patient

Acute Upper GI bleed Mx

Acute

Acute – ABCDE Approach & refer to senior + GI team
Oxygen via 15L non-rebreather if required
2 large wide bore cannulae

Definitive

Variceal Bleed

On admission: Terlipressin + prophylactic axbx
Post resus- Endoscopic band ligation

Calculate Rockall Rebleed score

Non- Variceal Bleed

Endoscopic thermal cautery/mechanical clipping
Post endoscopy- IV PPI

Calculate Rockall Rebleed score

Note on management framework:
For acute scenarios, acute & definitive
For chronic/long term mx: Conservative, Medical, Surgical

Peptic Uler Disease

Sore of the gastrointestinal lining

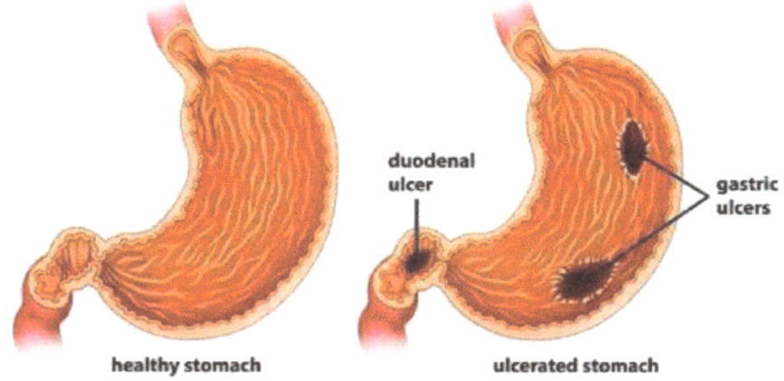

Aetiology

- H. pylori, NSAIDs, SSRIs

Signs and symptoms

- Epigastric pain, nausea
- If gastric- pain when eating; if duodenal- pain relived by eating
- Complications: Perforation, acute bleed

Investigations

- Urea breath test

Treatment

- If H pylori –ve- PPI
- If H pylori +ve- 321 eradication therapy
  (1 PPI + 2abx (amoxicillin and clarithromycin))

Station 2

Setting	**You are a 4th year medical student in the emergency department**
Patient details	**Colin, a 35 year old woman, presents with one week worsening of diarrhoea.**
Task	**Please take a 7 min history**

Station 2

35F
PC – Bloody diarrhoea

HPC
Change in bowel habits hx
Consistency- Diarrhoea
Colour- Red
Course- Intermittent over last year but much worse this week

Episodes- 10 per day

If blood, how much- not sure
Mixed with stools?- Yes

Abdo pain hx
SOCRATES-
Crampy lower abdominal pain, relieved by defecation

Travel history- went to spain 6 months ago

PMHx
Nil

FHx
Aunt had bowel problems

Systems review:
Nil gynaecology
Nil genitourinary
Nil neurological
Nil cardiovascular
Nil respiratory

DHx
Tried 2/7 amoxicillin when it first started but no relief

Social
Two children, both well

Smokes 10 per day
Rarely drinks

ICE:
Just wants it to stop

Differentials?

Differentials

Always give 3 – generally 2 of the most likely system involved and 1 of another

Looking at the patient demographic can give a clue but don't stereotype!

- **Ulcerative colitis**
- **Crohn's disease**
- **Ischaemic colitis**
- **Diverticulitis**

Inflammatory Bowel Disease

Chronic inflammation of the gastrointestinal tract

Crohn's

Patchy inflammation from mouth to anus

Non specific- Weight loss, lethargy
Abdominal pain

Diarrhoea (may be bloody)
Perianal disease e.g. skin tags, ulcers

Ulcerative colitis

Chronic inflammation from rectum to ileocecal calve

Bloody diarrhea
Urgency
Tenesmus
LLQ pain

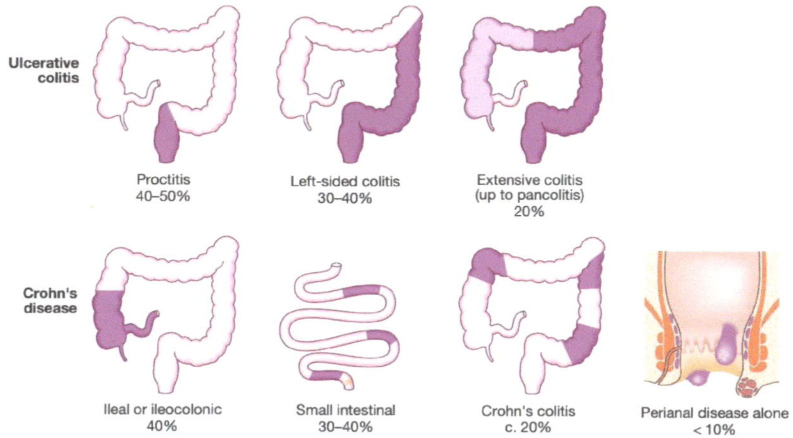

Fig. 21.45 Common patterns of disease distribution in inflammatory bowel disease.

Inflammatory Bowel Disease Ix

Bedside: Vital signs

Bloods: FBC, Inflammatory markers, pANCA, LFTs, stool analysis

Imaging: Abdominal X-ray; barium enema, colonoscopy (if in remission)

Special tests: For UC- Truelove and Witts' severity index

Crohn's disease Xray:
Kantor's string

Endoscopy: Skip lesions
Cobble stoning

Histology: Rose thorn ulcers
Inflammation through all layers
Increased goblet cells Granulomas

Ulcerative colitis Lead pipe colon

Red raw mucosa

No inflammation beyond submucosa Pseudopolyps
Crypt abscesses
Depleted goblet cells

Inflammatory Bowel Disease Ix

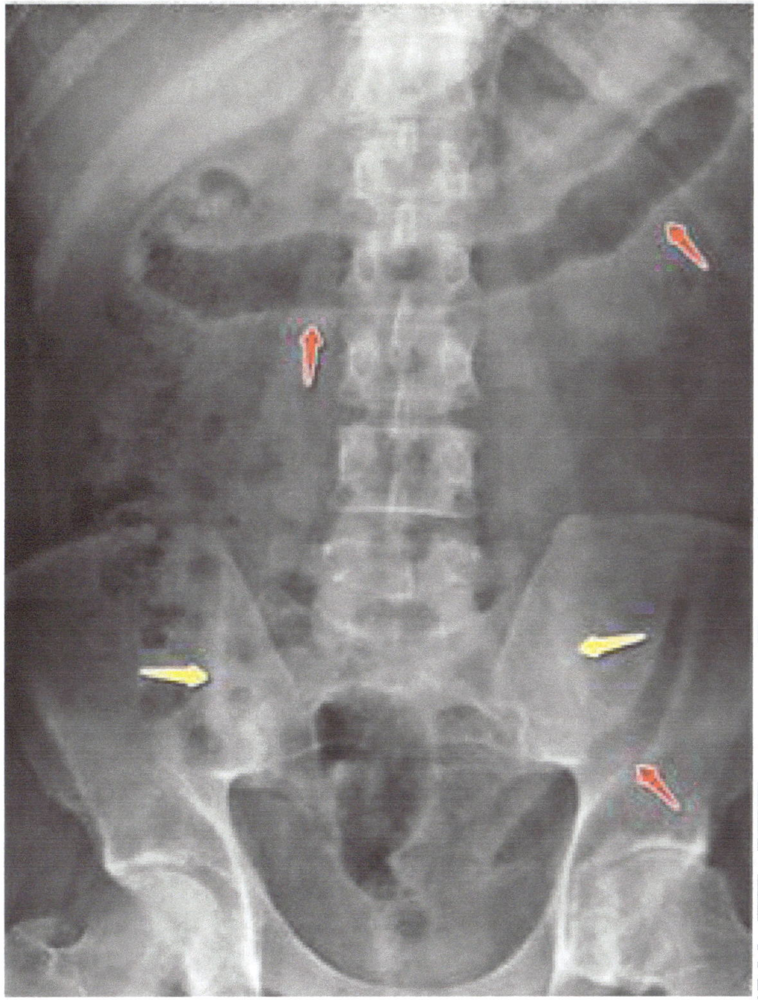

Abdominal X-ray:
Lead pipe colon
Ankylosis of left sacroiliac joint and partial ankylosis on right

Ulcerative Colitis

Inflammatory Bowel Disease Mx

Note on management framework:
For acute scenarios, acute & definitive
For chronic/long term mx: Conservative, Medical, Surgical

Ulcerative colitis

Acute

ABCDE – Senior
Stabilise the patient

Definitive Medical:
Mild-Moderate
5-ASA (mesalazine)

Severe Admit
+ IV steroids

Long term
Mild-Mod: 5-ASA
Severe- Mercaptopurine/Azathioprine

Crohn's Disease

Acute:
ABCDE – Senior Stabilise
the patient

Definitive
Mild flare- Oral prednisolone
Severe flare- IV and topical hydrocortisone

Long term:
Mercatopurine/Azathoprine

Consider surgical approach

Station 3

Setting	**You are a 4th year medical student in the GP surgery**
Patient details	**Aarija, a 56 year old woman presents complaining of abdominal pain**
Task	**Please take a focused 7 min history**

Station 3

1) Please could you summarise your history

On Examination:
Vital signs- 38.5 degrees (febrile), HR 108, BP 124/76
Normal cardioresp exam

Tender in RUQ and epigastrium with guarding and rebound tenderness

2) State your top 3 differentials.

3) Which investigations would you request in this patient?

Station 3

On Examination:

Vital signs- 38.5 degrees (febrile), HR 108, BP 124/76 Normal cardioresp exam

Tender in RUQ and epigastrium with guarding and rebound tenderness

		Normal ranges
Haemoglobin	14.7 g/dL	11.7–15.7 g/dL
White cell count	19.8 × 10^9/L	3.5–11.0 × 10^9/L
Platelets	239 × 10^9/L	150–440 × 10^9/L
Sodium	137 mmol/L	135–145 mmol/L
Potassium	4.8 mmol/L	3.5–5.0 mmol/L
Urea	8.6 mmol/L	2.5–6.7 mmol/L
Creatinine	116 μmol/L	70–120 μmol/L
Bilirubin	19 μmol/L	3–17 μmol/L
Alkaline phosphatase	58 IU/L	30–300 IU/L
Alanine aminotransferase (AAT)	67 IU/L	5–35 IU/L
Gamma-glutamyl transpeptidase	72 IU/L	11–51 IU/L
C-reactive protein (CRP)	256 mg/L	<5 mg/L

Differentials

- Acute cholecystitis
- Acute pancreatitis
- Abdominal aortic aneurysm

Gallstones and their progression

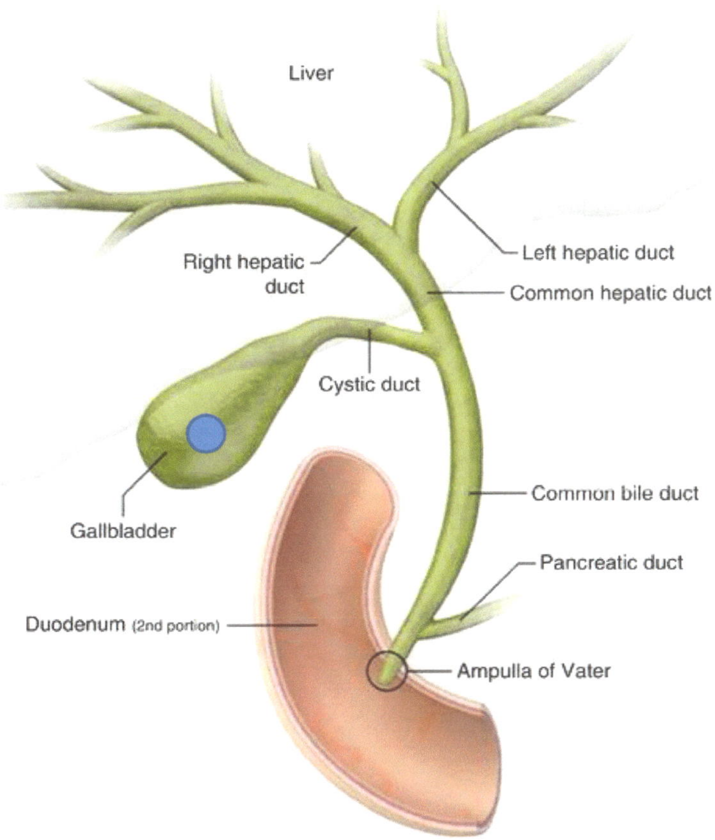

Cholelithiasis- Gall stones, 80% asymptomatic

Biliary colic- Episodic pain, worse after eating fatty meals

Gallstones and their progression

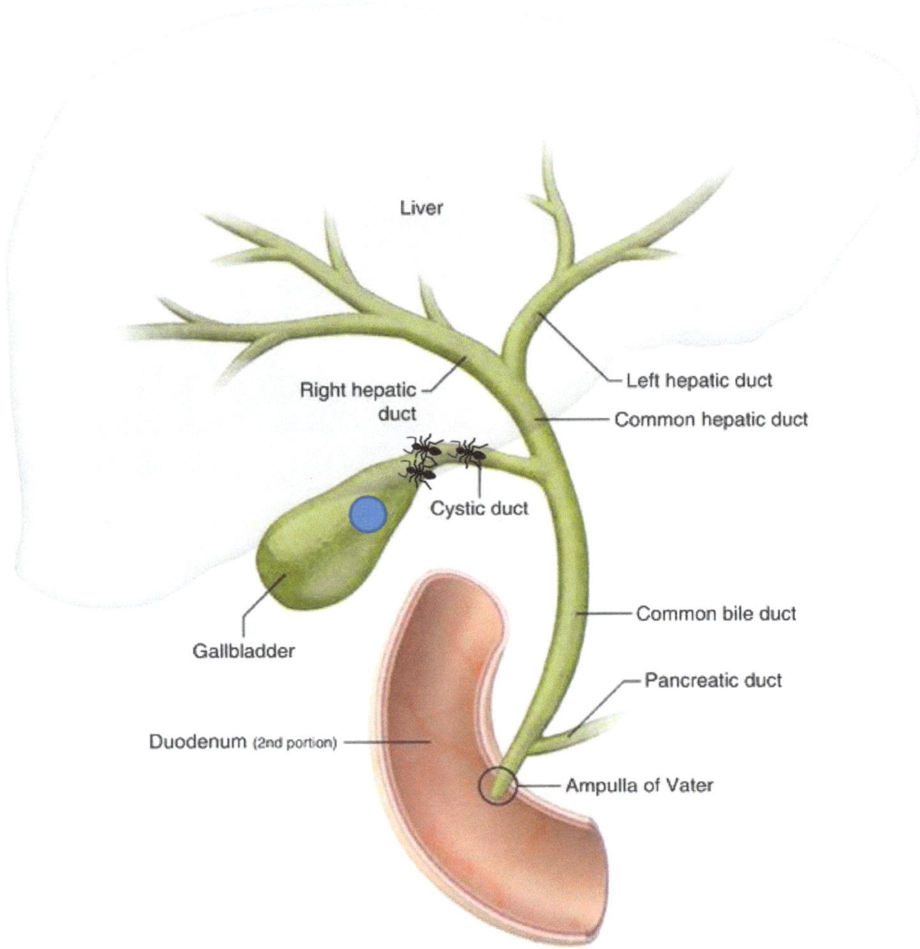

Cholelithiasis- Gall stones, 80% asymptomatic

Biliary colic- Episodic pain, worse after eating fatty meals

Acute cholecystitis- Gallbladder inflammation due to blocked cystic duct

Ascending cholangitis- Bacterial infection of bile duct=> Charcot's triad (jaundice, RUQ pain, fever)

Gallstones and their progression

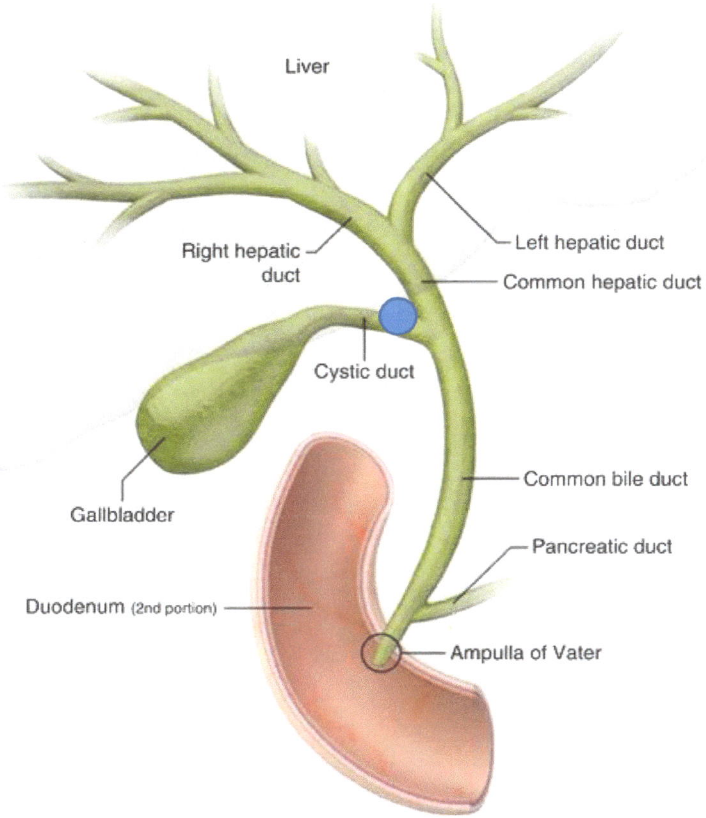

Cholelithiasis- Gall stones, 80% asymptomatic

Biliary colic- Episodic pain, worse after eating fatty meals

Acute cholecystitis- Gallbladder inflammation due to blocked cystic duct

Ascending cholangitis- Bacterial infection of bile duct=> Charcot's triad (jaundice, RUQ pain, fever)

Choledocholithiasis- Stone in CBD=> obstructive symptoms (dark urine, pale stools)

Biliary Tree Ix

Bedside: Observations

Bloods: FBC, LFT, Amylase

Imaging: CXR

Special tests: *US*, ERCP

MRCP (if difficult to visualise US)

Framework for investigations:
BBOXES: Bedside, bloods, orifices, xrays, ?everything else, special tests
Bedside, bloods, imaging, special tests

Acute cholecystitis Mx

Acute

ABCDE approach

Refer to seniors + GI surgeons Give pain relief

Consider IV broad spectrum antibiotics Prepare

for surgery- NBM, medication review

Definitive

Laparoscopic cholecystectomy

Note on management framework:
For acute scenarios, acute & definitive
For chronic/long term mx: Conservative, Medical, Surgical

Station 4

Setting You are a 4th year medical student in the GP

Patient details Jean, a 74 year old female presents with intermittent lower abdominal pain.

Task Please take a focused 7 min history

Station 4

74F
PC – Lower abdominal pain

HoPC
Pain hx
S: LLQ
O: 10 years, worse over last week C: sometimes sharp
R:none
A: Distension in LIF, anorexia
T: Continuous; was previously colicky E: Relieved on defecation
S: 8/10 pain

Bowel habits hx
Consistency- constipation, small hard pieces; has not opened for 2 days Colour- Normal
Course- Constant constipation

An episode of blood 4 years ago- had barium enema

PMHx
Hysterectomy for fibroids (2003)

DHx
None

FHx
IHD
T2DM

SH
Non smoker Non drinker Lives alone
Independent

ICE:
Thinks it might have something to do with previous x-ray

Differentials?

Differentials

- Diverticulitis
- Endometriosis
- Colorectal cancer

Diverticulitis

Inflamed outpouching of bowel wall

Diverticulosis=Outpouching between taenia colon

RF: Age + low fibre diet

Symptoms: Altered bowel habits, colicky left sided abdo pain, bloody stools

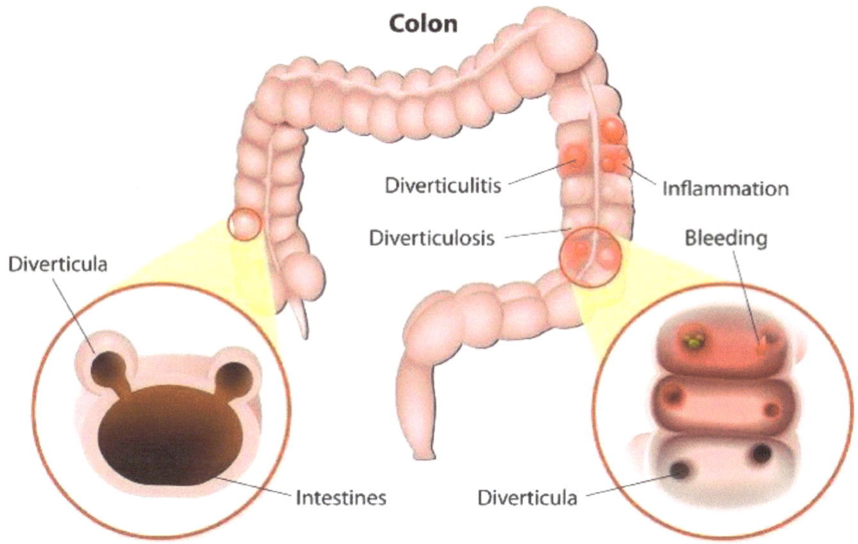

<u>Diverticulitis</u>

Acute onset, severe abdominal pain
Usually LLQ
Usually Constipation
PR bleeding

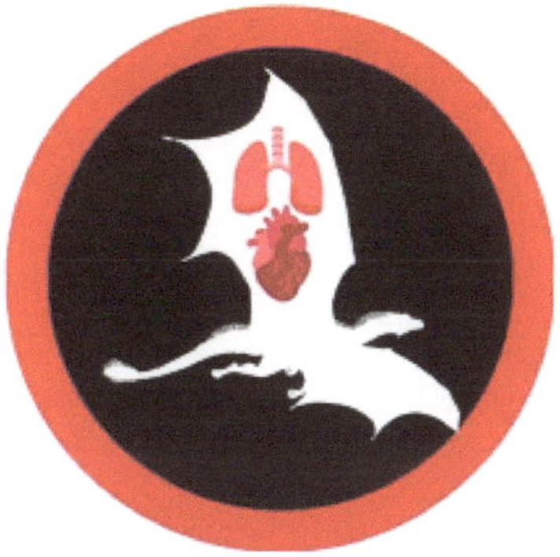

Diverticulitis Ix

Bedside: Observations

Bloods: FBC, U&E, CRP

Imaging: CT

Special tests: Colonoscopy (avoid initially due to risk of perforation)

Diverticulitis Mx

Acute

A-E approach Alert

seniors

Definitive

Uncomplicated

Supportive

Antibiotics e.g. oral metronidazole + oral ceftriaxone

Complicated

Broad spectrum IV abx

If IV abx insufficient :

Abscess- if no signs of improvements with abx, percutaneous drainage

Perforation- emergency surgery (colectomy/Hartmann's)

Consider elective colectomy after resolution

Station 5

Setting	**You are a 4th** year medical student in the emergency department
Patient details	**22 year old woman presents complaining of tiredness**
Task	**Please take a focused 7 min history**

Station 5

1) **Please could you summarise your history and state your top 3 differentials.**

2) **Which investigations would you request in this patient?**

	Investigations		
			Normal
Haemoglobin		9.8 g/dL	11.7–15.7 g/dL
Mean corpuscular volume (MCV)		98 fL	80–99 fL
White cell count		6.5 × 10^9/L	3.5–11.0 × 10^9/L
Platelets		247 × 10^9/L	150–440 × 10^9/L
Red cell folate		44 mg/L	>160 mg/L
Vitamin B_{12}		280 ng/L	176–925 ng/L
Thyroid-stimulating hormone		3.5 mU/L	0.3–6.0 mU/L
Free thyroxine		12.9 pmol/L	9.0–22.0 pmol/L
The blood film is reported as a dimorphic film with remnants of nuclear material (Howell–Jolly bodies) in some of the red blood cells.			

Differentials

- Coeliac disease
- Small intestinal bacterial overgrowth
- IBS

Coellac Disease

Insensitivity to gluten

Signs and symptoms

Chronic/intermittent steatorrhea
Failure to thrive
Unexplained GI symptoms

Macrocytic anaemia (folate/B12 deficiency)

Complications

Anaemia
Hyposplenism (=> Howell-Jolly bodies)
Osteoporosis
Lactose intolerance
T cell lymphoma

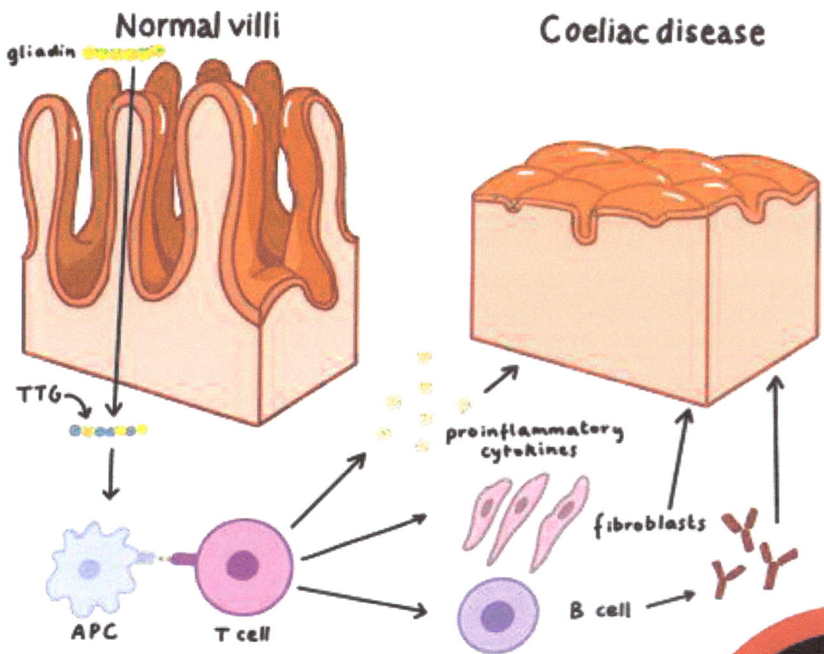

Coeliac disease Ix

Bedside: Observations

Bloods: FBC

Imaging: Small bowel endoscopy, small bowel histology

Special tests: tTG & IgA

Coeliac disease Mx

Conservative

Gluten free diet

Medical

Vitamin and mineral supplementation

Surgical

Nil

Note on management framework:
For acute scenarios, acute & definitive
For chronic/long term mx: Conservative, Medical, Surgical

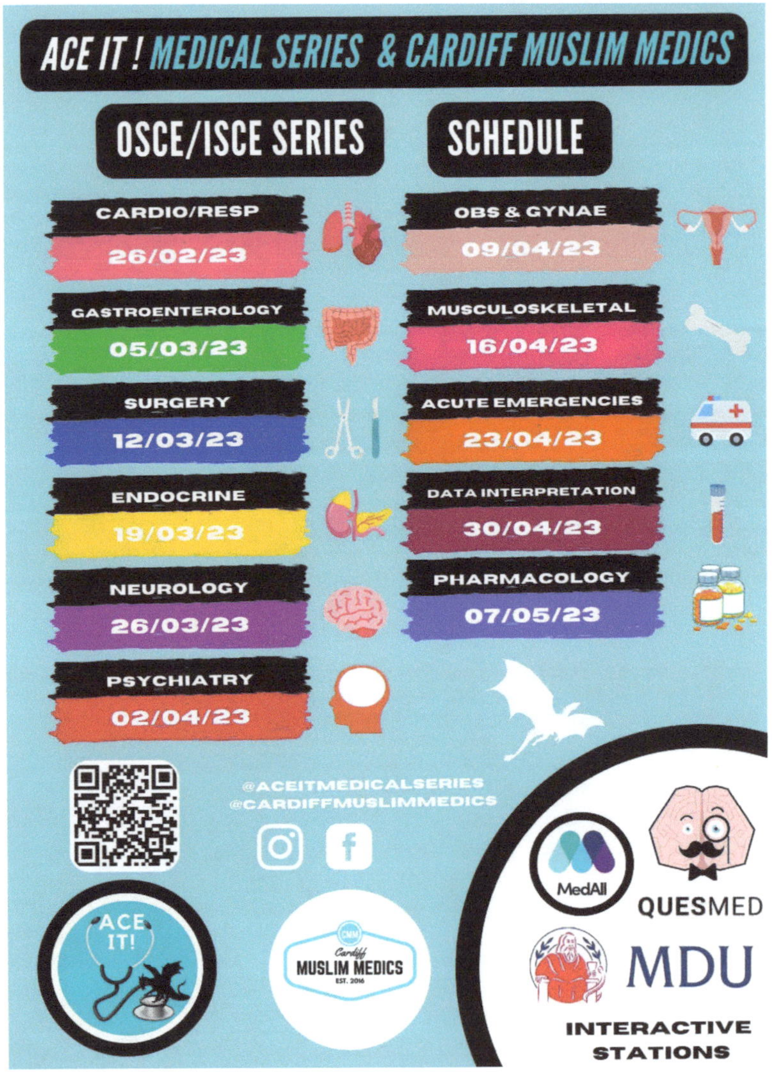

THANK YOU FOR LISTENING! 😊

ANY QUESTIONS?

FEEDBACK FORM FOR SLIDES

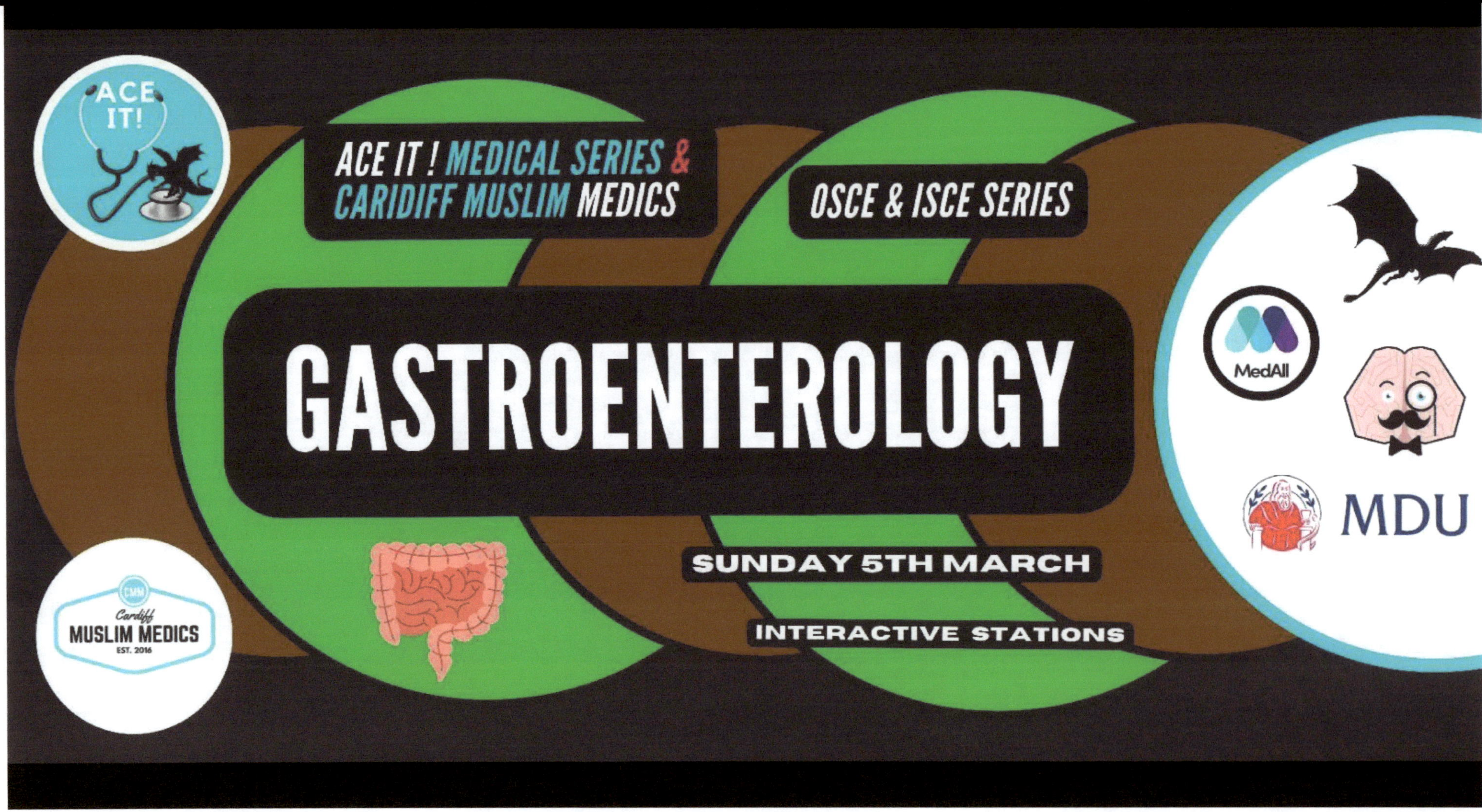
ACE IT!
ACE IT ! MEDICAL SERIES & CARIDIFF MUSLIM MEDICS
OSCE & ISCE SERIES
GASTROENTEROLOGY
SUNDAY 5TH MARCH
INTERACTIVE STATIONS
CMM
Cardiff
MUSLIM MEDICS
EST. 2016
MedAll
MDU

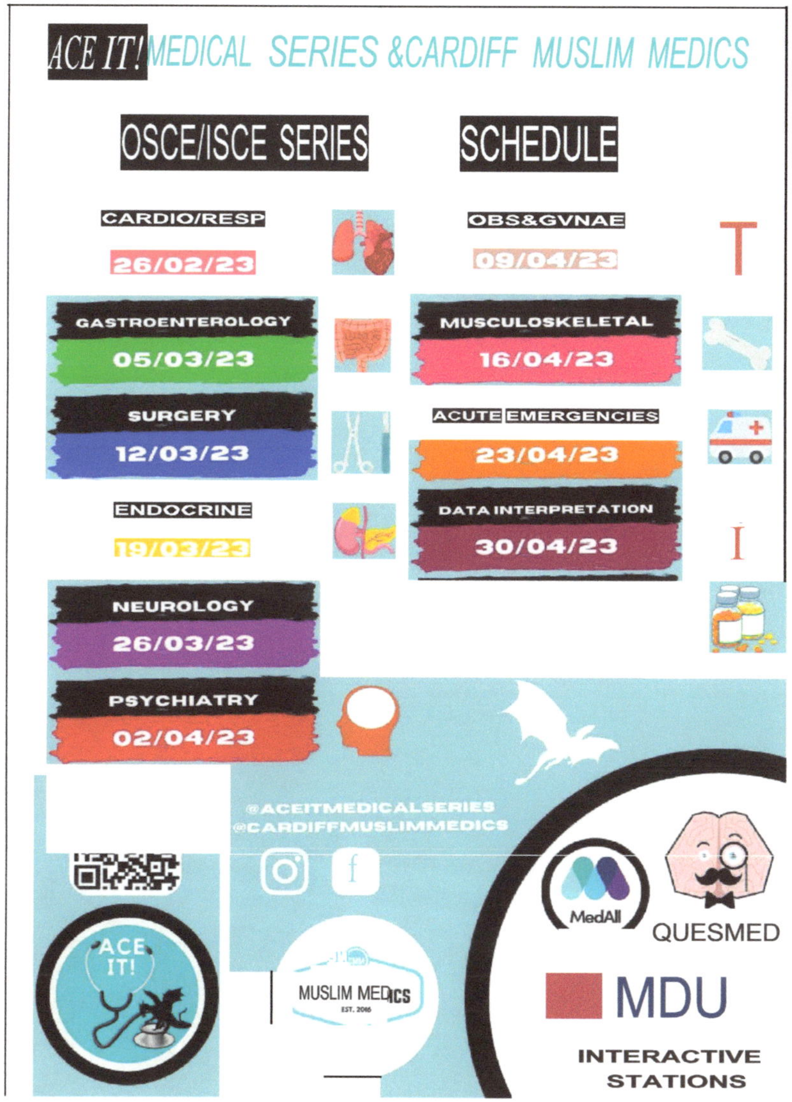
ACE IT! MEDICAL SERIES & CARDIFF MUSLIM MEDICS
OSCE/ISCE SERIES
SCHEDULE
CARDIO/RESP
26/02/23
GASTROENTEROLOGY
05/03/23
SURGERY
12/03/23
ENDOCRINE
19/03/23
NEUROLOGY
26/03/23
PSYCHIATRY
02/04/23
OBS&GYNAE
09/04/23
MUSCULOSKELETAL
16/04/23
ACUTE EMERGENCIES
23/04/23
DATA INTERPRETATION
30/04/23
@ACEITMEDICALSERIES
@CARDIFFMUSLIMMEDICS
ACE IT!
MUSLIM MEDICS
MedAll
QUESMED
MDU
INTERACTIVE STATIONS

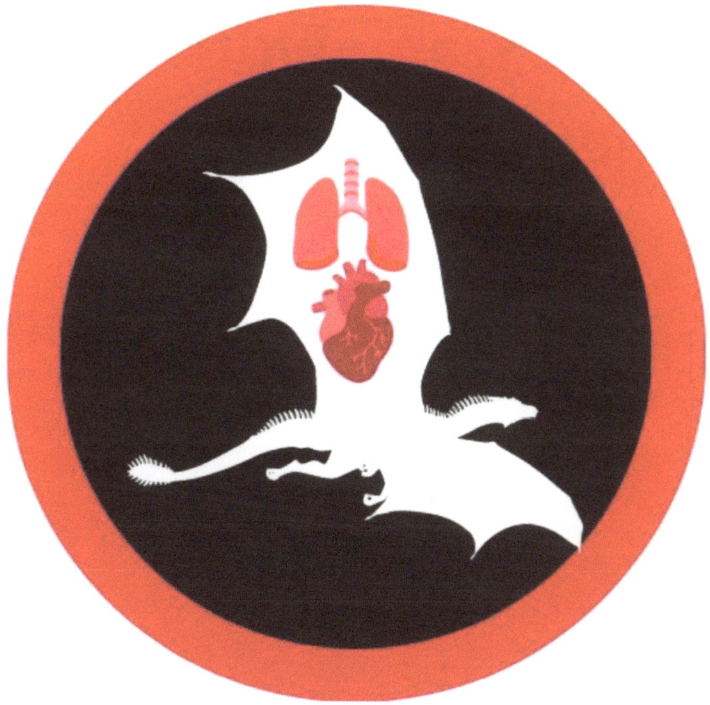

Learning Outcomes

To practice taking GI histories

To develop a framework for summaries and ongoing management plans

To revise some common GI conditions
(hidden for the sake of the cases)

Symptom explosions GI History

1) ABDOMINAL PAIN

SOCRATES
Site=organ

Travel/diet history

2) CHANGE IN BOWEL HABITS

Consistency
Colour
Course

If blood, how much and ?mixed with stools

Travel/diet history

3) VOMITING

Content- ?blood
Colour
Amount
Episodes

4) WEIGHT LOSS

How much?
Dress/clothes sizes, comments from others

How long? *>5% 6-12 months*

Intentional or unintentional

5) HAEMODYNAMIC COMPROMISE

Pale, light headed, dizzy, syncope, drowsy
Racing heart

Could indicate serious pathology

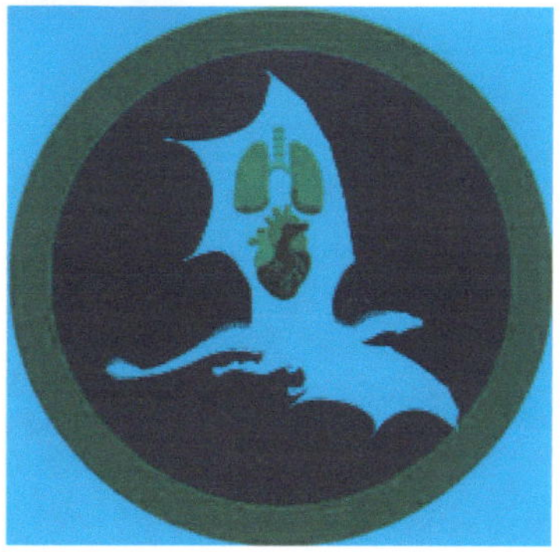

If female patient- take a brief obs and gynae overview (see next slide)

Upper GI paln History

1. PC
2. HoPC – **SOCRATES, change in bowel habits; if female, do a brief obs&gynae review**
   BSc MS: Births, Sexual history, Contraception, Menstruation, Smears
3. PMH/PSH- **Abdominal surgeries (=> adhesions)**
4. DHx – **Allergies!! Current medications and OTC (nb NSAIDs)**
5. FHx – **any GI conditions or cancers**
6. Social – **Travel/diet history, smoking, ALCOHOL, etc**
7. ICE
8. Systems review- **Top to toe**

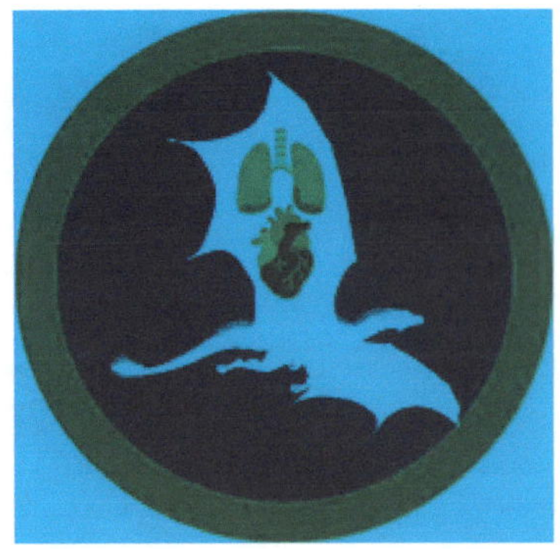

In 4 min Hx for acute stations, key points are PC HPC + DHx should you run out of time

Some GI differentials to have in mind

1) STOMACH

Peptic ulcer disease
Gastroenteritis Gastric cancer

2) OESOPHAGUS

GORD
- Oesophagitis
- Barret's

Oesophageal cancer
Pharyngeal pouch
Achalasia
Varices

3) PANCREAS

Acute pancreatitis
Chronic pancreatitis
Pancreatic cancer

4) BILIARY TREE

Biliary colic
Acute cholecystitis
Ascending cholangitis
Cholangiocarcinoma

5) SMALL INTESTINE (+Others)

Inferior MI
Abdominal Aortic Aneurysm
Acute mesenteric ischaemia
Ischaemic colitis

IBD (UC/Crohn's)
Coeliac's

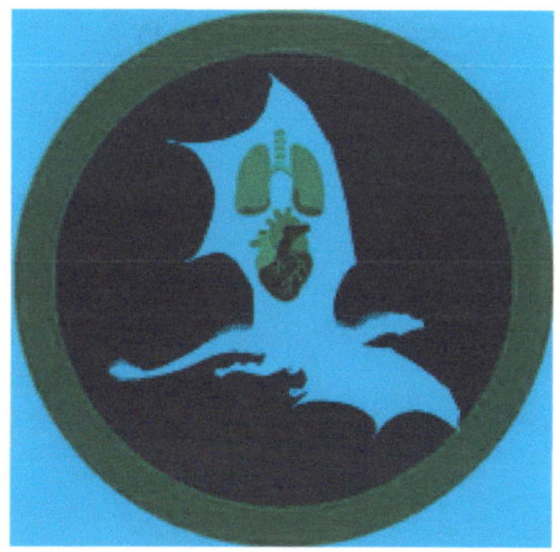

Surgical Sieve

Question 1:Which system?
Question 2:Which organ?
Question 3:Which process?

Vitamin CDEF
Vascular
Inflammatory/infection
Trauma
Autoimmune
Metabolic
Iatrogenic
Neoplastic
Congenital
Drugs
Endocrine
Functional

Question 4:Why?

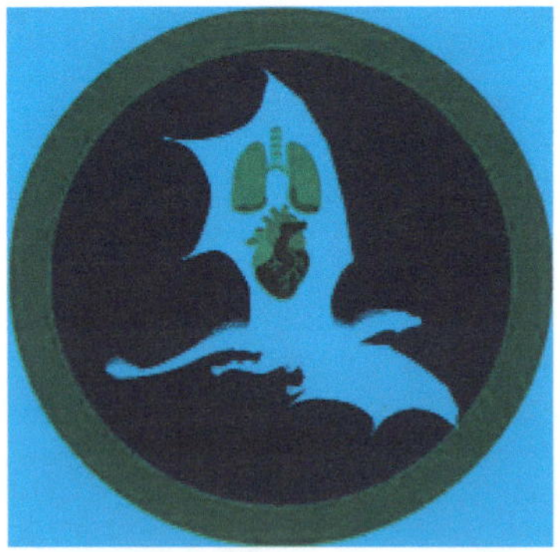

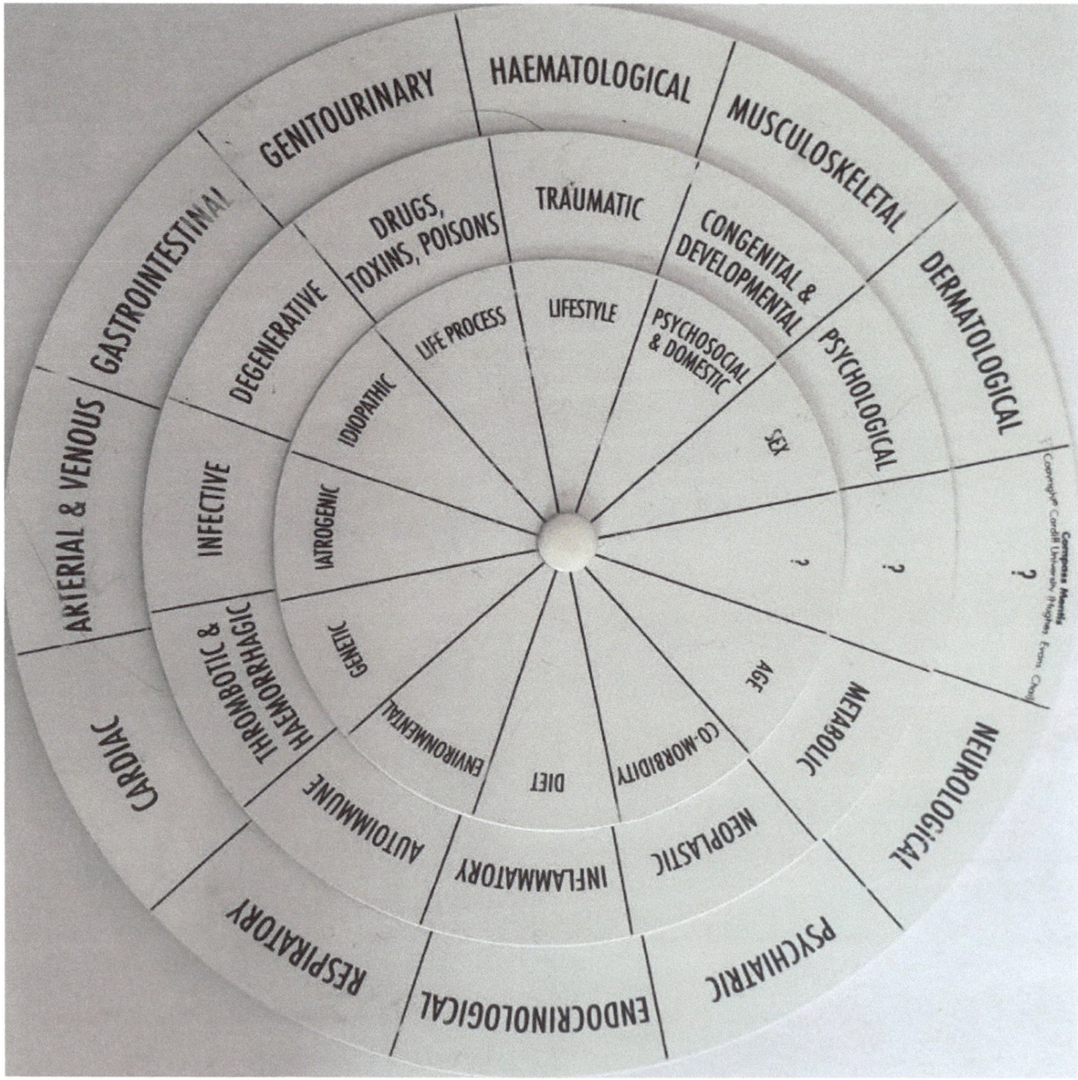

Station 1

Setting	**You are a 4th year medical student in the emergency department**
Patient details	**Yusuf a 52-year-old gentleman presents after vomiting fresh red blood.**
Task	**Please take a 4 min history**

Station 1

1) Please could you summarise your history and state your top 3 differentials.

Summary:

Patient name, age and presenting complaint

Follow history structure

Mention relevant positive findings Important negatives

Differentials

2) Which investigations would you request in this patient?

Differentials

Always give 3 – generally 2 of the most likely system involved and 1 of another

Looking at the patient demographic can give a clue but don't stereotype!

- **Acute Upper GI bleed**
- **Variceal bleed Peptic**
- **ulcer disease Mallory**
- **Weiss Tear**

Acute Upper GI bleed

Bleeding from the gastrointestinal tract proximal to the duodenum

Causes

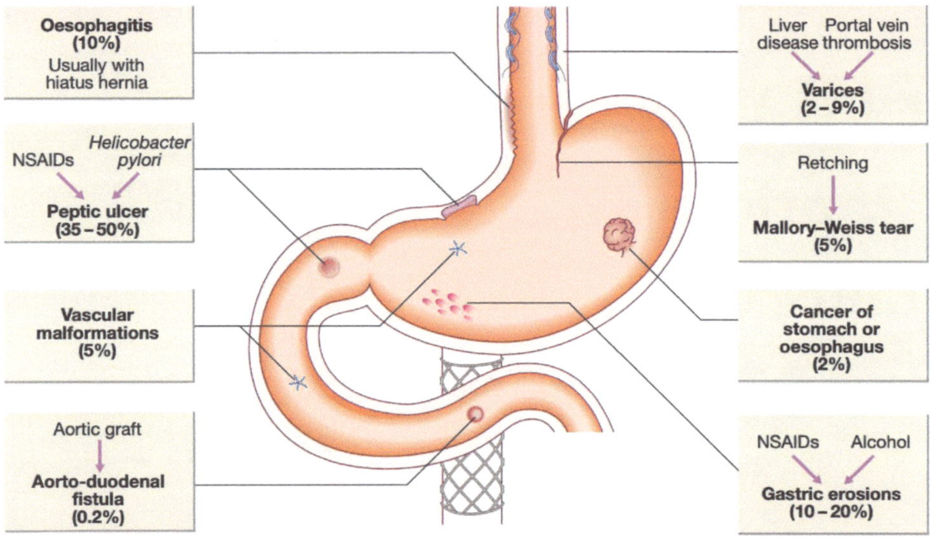

Fig. 21.19 Causes of acute upper gastrointestinal haemorrhage. Frequency is given in parentheses. (NSAIDs = non-steroidal anti-inflammatory drugs)

Symptoms

Haematemesis

Melaena

Symptoms of blood loss

Acute Upper GI bleed

Key Investigations

Bedside-

Blatchford bleeding score

Used on admission to estimate need for intervention

Vital signs

Bloods- FBC, U&E, LFT,
Coagulation screen, crossmatch + G&S

Imaging- Endoscopy (w/i 24h, immediate if severe)

Framework for investigations:
BBOXES: Bedside, bloods, orifices, xrays, ?everything else, special tests
Bedside, bloods, imaging, special tests

Acute Upper GI bleed Ix

Endoscopic image Name: X
DOB: 09-09-1971

Taken 05/03/2023

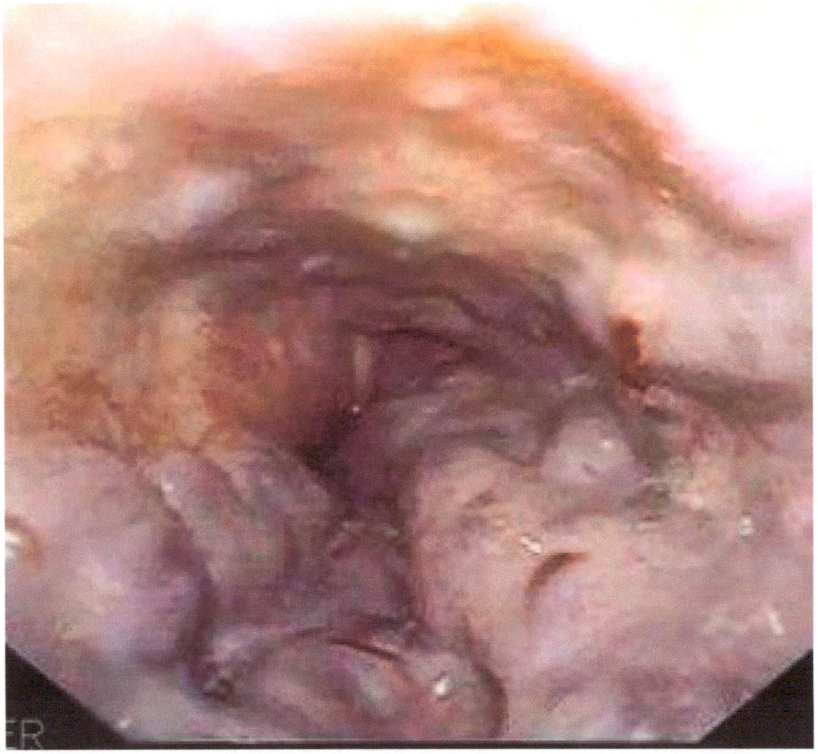

Please interpret the image above and formulate a management plan for the patient

Acute Upper GI bleed Mx

Acute

Acute – ABCDE Approach & refer to senior + GI team
Oxygen via 15L non-rebreather if required
2 large wide bore cannulae

Definitive

Variceal Bleed

On admission: Terlipressin + prophylactic axbx
Post resus- Endoscopic band ligation

Calculate Rockall Rebleed score

Non- Variceal Bleed

Endoscopic thermal cautery/mechanical clipping
Post endoscopy- IV PPI

Calculate Rockall Rebleed score

Note on management framework:
For acute scenarios, acute & definitive
For chronic/long term mx: Conservative, Medical, Surgical

Peptic Ulcer Disease

Sore of the gastrointestinal lining

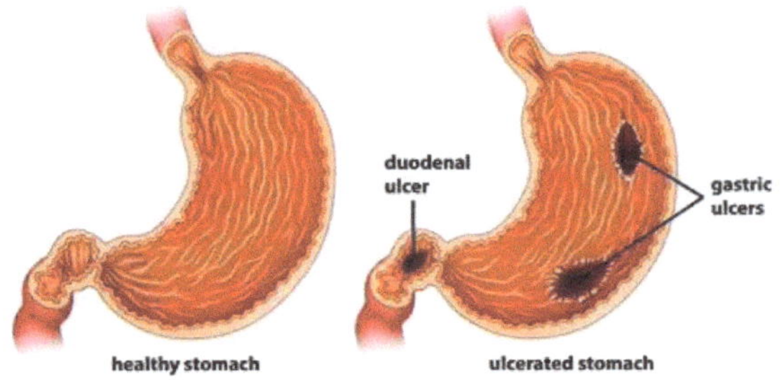

Aetiology

- H. pylori, NSAIDs, SSRIs

Signs and symptoms

- Epigastric pain, nausea
- If gastric- pain when eating; if duodenal- pain relived by eating
- Complications: Perforation, acute bleed

Investigations

- Urea breath test

Treatment

- If H pylori –ve- PPI
- If H pylori +ve- 321 eradication therapy
  (1 PPI + 2abx (amoxicillin and clarithromycin))

Station 2

Setting	**You are a 4th year medical student in the emergency department**
Patient details	**Colin, a 35 year old woman, presents with one week worsening of diarrhoea.**
Task	**Please take a 7 min history**

Station 2

35F
PC – Bloody diarrhoea

HPC
Change in bowel habits hx
Consistency- Diarrhoea
Colour- Red
Course- Intermittent over last year but much worse this week

Episodes- 10 per day

If blood, how much- not sure
Mixed with stools?- Yes

Abdo pain hx
SOCRATES-
Crampy lower abdominal pain, relieved by defecation

Travel history- went to spain 6 months ago

PMHx
Nil

FHx
Aunt had bowel problems

Systems review:
Nil gynaecology
Nil genitourinary
Nil neurological
Nil cardiovascular
Nil respiratory

DHx
Tried 2/7 amoxicillin when it first started but no relief

Social
Two children, both well

Smokes 10 per day
Rarely drinks

ICE:
Just wants it to stop

Differentials?

Differentials

Always give 3 – generally 2 of the most likely system involved and 1 of another

Looking at the patient demographic can give a clue but don't stereotype!

- Ulcerative colitis
- Crohn's disease
- Ischaemic colitis
- Diverticulitis

Inflammatory Bowel Disease

Chronic inflammation of the gastrointestinal tract

Crohn's

Patchy inflammation from mouth to anus

Non specific- Weight loss, lethargy
Abdominal pain
Diarrhoea (may be bloody) Perianal disease e.g. skin tags, ulcers

Ulcerative colitis

Chronic inflammation from rectum to ileocecal calve

Bloody diarrhoea Urgency Tenesmus
LLQ pain

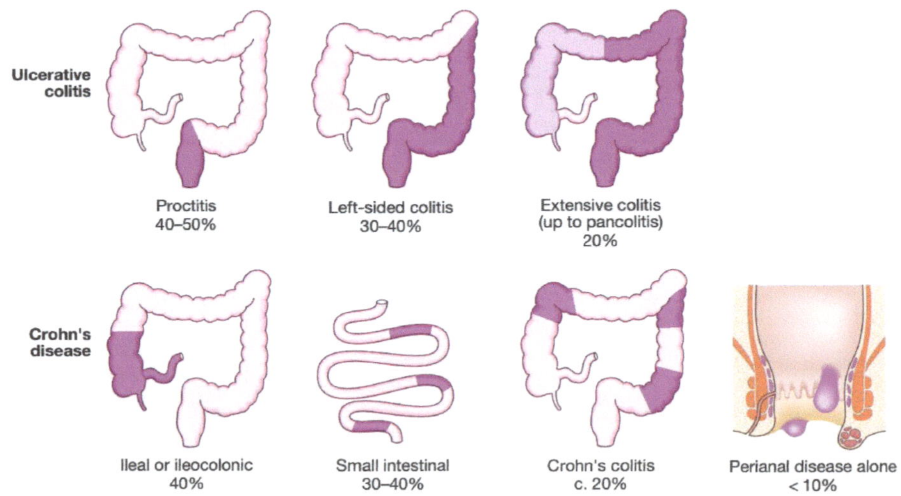

Fig. 21.45 Common patterns of disease distribution in inflammatory bowel disease.

Inflammatory Bowel Disease Ix

Bedside: Vital signs

Bloods: FBC, Inflammatory markers, pANCA, LFTs, stool analysis

Imaging: Abdominal X-ray; barium enema, colonoscopy (if in remission)

Special tests: For UC- Truelove and Witts' severity index

Crohn's disease Xray:
Kantor's string

Endoscopy: Skip lesions
Cobble stoning

Histology: Rose thorn ulcers
Inflammation through all layers
Increased goblet cells Granulomas

Ulcerative colitis Lead pipe colon

Red raw mucosa

No inflammation beyond submucosa Pseudopolyps
Crypt abscesses
Depleted goblet cells

Inflammatory Bowel Disease Ix

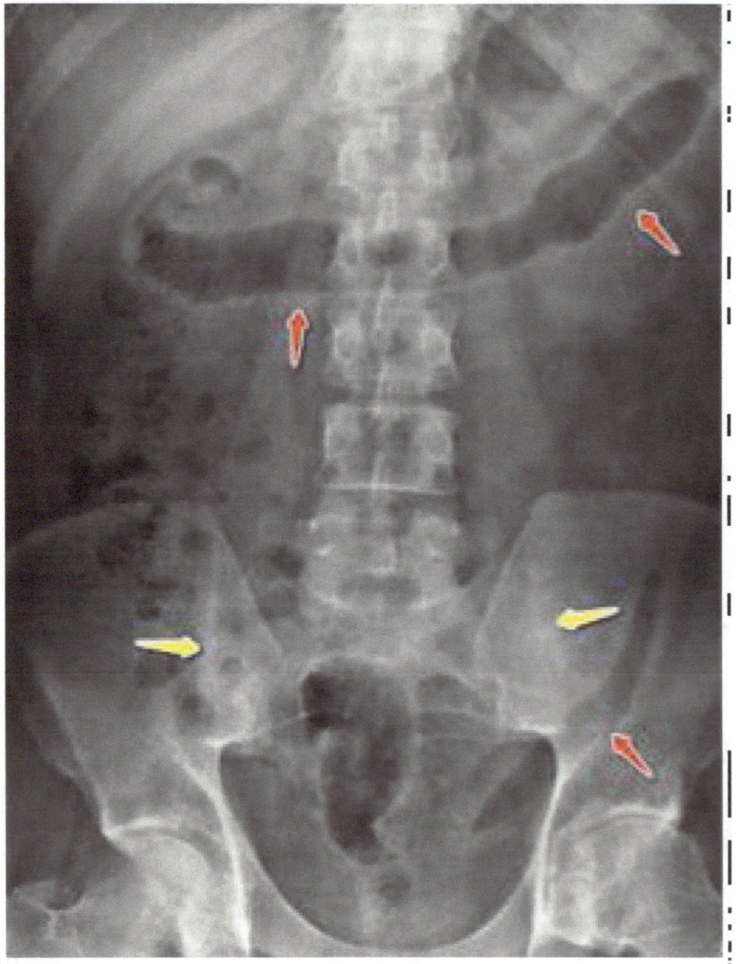

Ulcerative Colitis

Abdominal X-ray:
Lead pipe colon
Ankylosis of left sacroiliac joint and partial ankylosis on right

Inflammatory Bowel Disease Mx

Note on management framework:
For acute scenarios, acute & definitive
For chronic/long term mx: Conservative, Medical, Surgical

Ulcerative colitis

Acute

ABCDE – Senior
Stabilise the patient

Definitive Medical:
Mild-Moderate
5-ASA (mesalazine)

Severe Admit
+ IV steroids

Long term
Mild-Mod: 5-ASA
Severe- Mercaptopurine/Azathioprine

Crohn's Disease

Acute:

ABCDE – Senior
Stabilise the patient

Definitive
Mild flare- Oral prednisolone Severe flare- IV and topical hydrocortisone

Long term:
Mercatopurine/Azathoprine

Consider surgical approach

Station 3

Setting	**You are a 4th year medical student in the GP surgery**
Patient details	**Aarija, a 56 year old woman presents complaining of abdominal pain**
Task	**Please take a focused 7 min history**

Station 3

1) Please could you summarise your history

On Examination:
Vital signs- 38.5 degrees (febrile), HR 108, BP 124/76 Normal cardioresp exam
Tender in RUQ and epigastrium with guarding and rebound tenderness

2) State your top 3 differentials.

3) Which investigations would you request in this patient?

Station 3

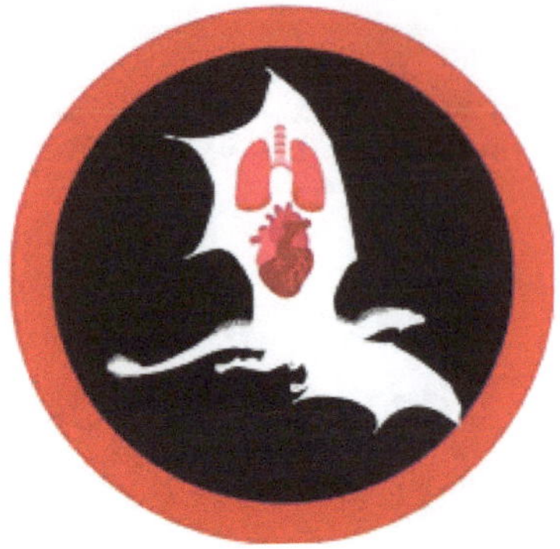

On Examination:

Vital signs- 38.5 degrees (febrile), HR 108, BP 124/76 Normal cardioresp exam

Tender in RUQ and epigastrium with guarding and rebound tenderness

		Normal ranges
Haemoglobin	14.7 g/dL	11.7–15.7 g/dL
White cell count	19.8 × 109/L	3.5–11.0 × 109/L
Platelets	239 × 109/L	150–440 × 109/L
Sodium	137 mmol/L	135–145 mmol/L
Potassium	4.8 mmol/L	3.5–5.0 mmol/L
Urea	8.6 mmol/L	2.5–6.7 mmol/L
Creatinine	116 μmol/L	70–120 μmol/L
Bilirubin	19 μmol/L	3–17 μmol/L
Alkaline phosphatase	58 IU/L	30–300 IU/L
Alanine aminotransferase (AAT)	67 IU/L	5–35 IU/L
Gamma-glutamyl transpeptidase	72 IU/L	11–51 IU/L
C-reactive protein (CRP)	256 mg/L	<5 mg/L

Differentials

- Acute cholecystitis
- Acute pancreatitis
- Abdominal aortic aneurysm

Gallstones and their progression

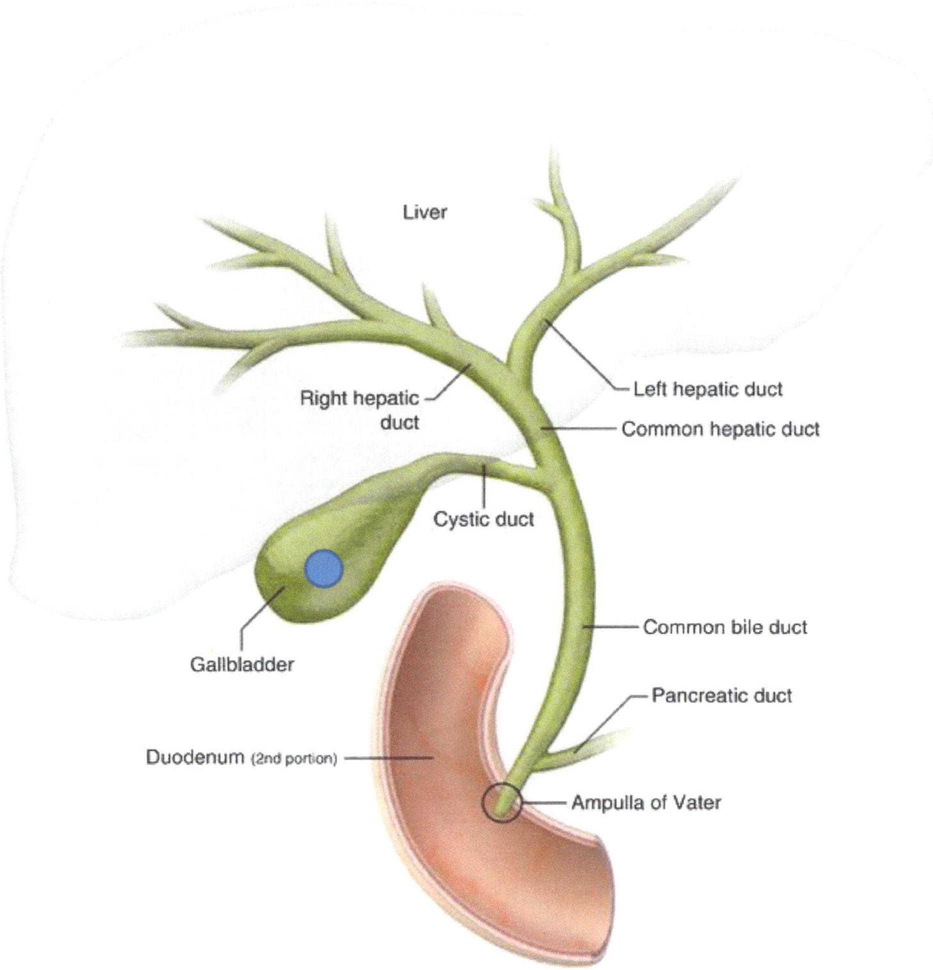

Cholelithiasis- Gall stones, 80% asymptomatic

Biliary colic- Episodic pain, worse after eating fatty meals

Gallstones and their progression

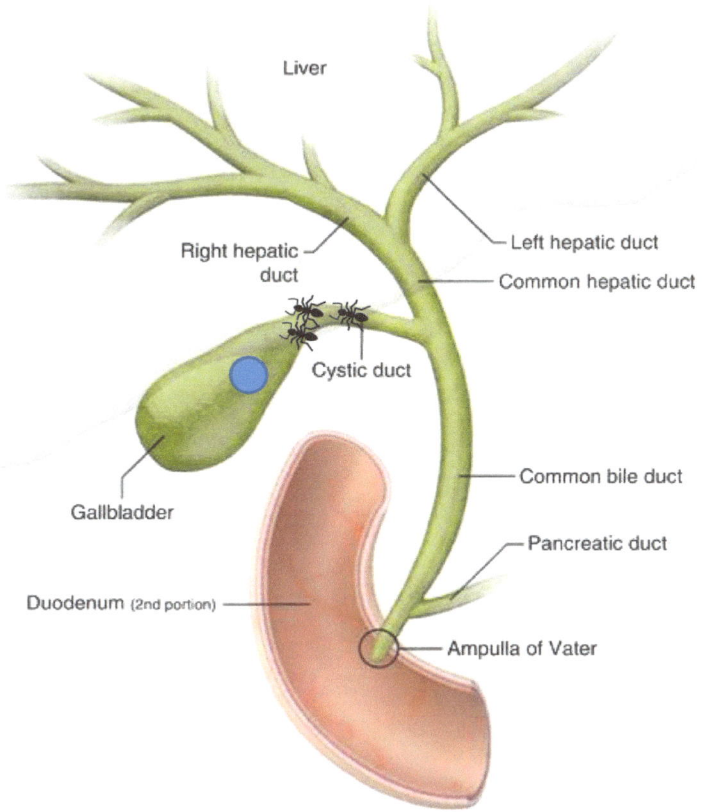

Cholelithiasis- Gall stones, 80% asymptomatic

Biliary colic- Episodic pain, worse after eating fatty meals

Acute cholecystitis- Gallbladder inflammation due to blocked cystic duct

Ascending cholangitis- Bacterial infection of bile duct=> Charcot's triad (jaundice, RUQ pain, fever)

Gallstones and their progression

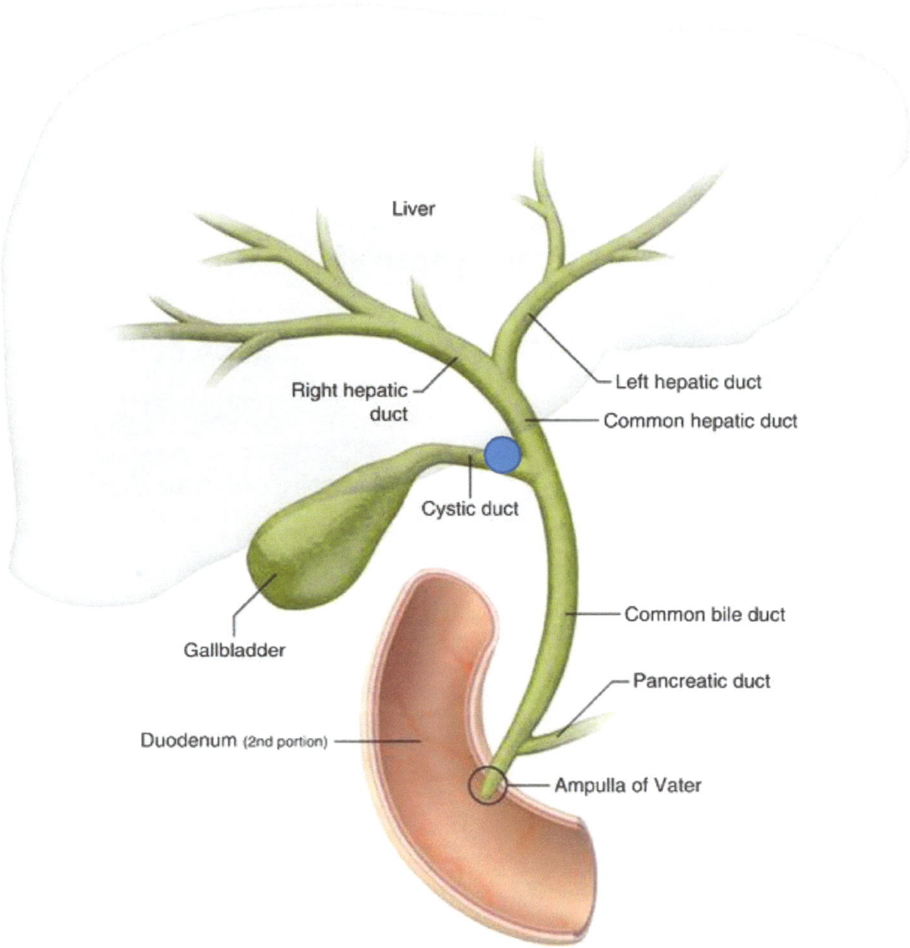

Cholelithiasis- Gall stones, 80% asymptomatic

Biliary colic- Episodic pain, worse after eating fatty meals

Acute cholecystitis- Gallbladder inflammation due to blocked cystic duct

Ascending cholangitis- Bacterial infection of bile duct=> Charcot's triad (jaundice, RUQ pain, fever)

Choledocholithiasis- Stone in CBD=> obstructive symptoms (dark urine, pale stools)

Biliary Tree Ix

Bedside: Observations

Bloods: FBC, LFT, Amylase

Imaging: CXR

Special tests: *US*, ERCP

MRCP (if difficult to visualise US)

Framework for investigations:
BBOXES: Bedside, bloods, orifices, xrays, ?everything else, special tests
Bedside, bloods, imaging, special tests

Acute cholecystitis Mx

Acute

ABCDE approach

Refer to seniors + GI surgeons

Give pain relief

Consider IV broad spectrum antibiotics

Prepare for surgery- NBM, medication review

Definitive

Laparoscopic cholecystectomy

Note on management framework:
For acute scenarios, acute & definitive
For chronic/long term mx: Conservative, Medical, Surgical

Station 4

Setting You are a 4th year medical student in the GP

Patient details Jean, a 74 year old female presents with intermittent lower abdominal pain.

Task Please take a focused 7 min history

Station 4

74F
PC – Lower abdominal pain

HoPC
Pain hx
S: LLQ
O: 10 years, worse over last week C: sometimes sharp
R:none
A: Distension in LIF, anorexia
T: Continuous; was previously colicky E: Relieved on defecation
S: 8/10 pain

Bowel habits hx
Consistency- constipation, small hard pieces; has not opened for 2 days Colour- Normal
Course- Constant constipation

An episode of blood 4 years ago- had barium enema

PMHx
Hysterectomy for fibroids (2003)

DHx
None

FHx
IHD
T2DM

SH
Non smoker
Non drinker
Lives alone
Independent

ICE:
Thinks it might have something to do with previous x-ray

Differentials?

Differentials

- Diverticulitis
- Endometriosis
- Colorectal cancer

Diverticulitis

Inflamed outpouching of bowel wall

Diverticulosis=Outpouching between taenia colon

RF: Age + low fibre diet

Symptoms: Altered bowel habits, colicky left sided abdo pain, bloody stools

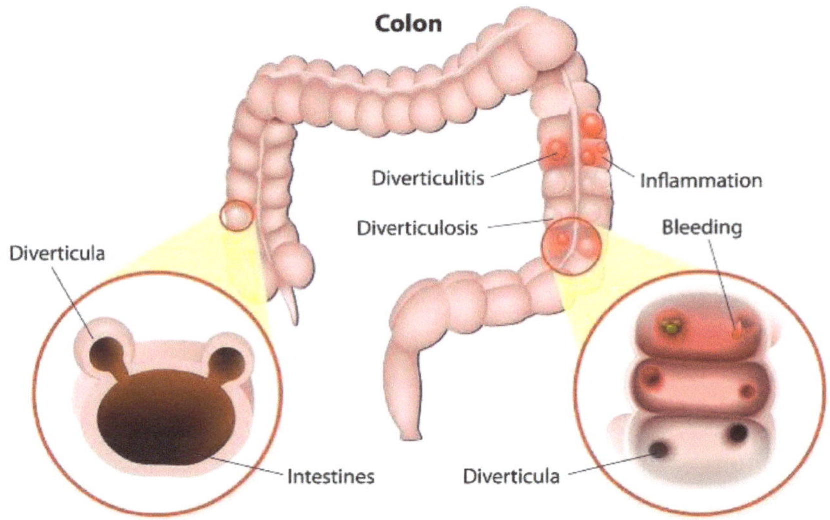

<u>Diverticulitis</u>

Acute onset, severe abdominal pain Usually LLQ

Usually Constipation PR bleeding

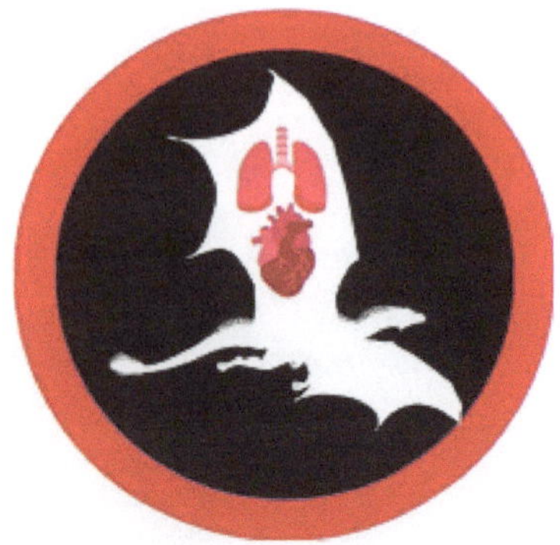

Diverticulitis Ix

Bedside: Observations

Bloods: FBC, U&E, CRP

Imaging: CT

Special tests: Colonoscopy (avoid initially due to risk of perforation)

Diverticulitis Mx

Acute

A-E approach Alert
seniors

Definitive

Uncomplicated

Supportive

Antibiotics e.g. oral metronidazole + oral ceftriaxone

Complicated

Broad spectrum IV abx

If IV abx insufficient :

Abscess- if no signs of improvements with abx, percutaneous drainage

Perforation- emergency surgery (colectomy/Hartmann's)

Consider elective colectomy after resolution

Station 5

Setting	**You are a 4th** year medical student in the emergency department
Patient details	**22 year old woman presents complaining of tiredness**
Task	**Please take a focused 7 min history**

Station 5

1) Please could you summarise your history and state your top 3 differentials.

2) Which investigations would you request in this patient?

	Investigations		
			Normal
Haemoglobin		9.8 g/dL	11.7–15.7 g/dL
Mean corpuscular volume (MCV)		98 fL	80–99 fL
White cell count		6.5 × 10^9/L	3.5–11.0 × 10^9/L
Platelets		247 × 10^9/L	150–440 × 10^9/L
Red cell folate		44 mg/L	>160 mg/L
Vitamin B_{12}		280 ng/L	176–925 ng/L
Thyroid-stimulating hormone		3.5 mU/L	0.3–6.0 mU/L
Free thyroxine		12.9 pmol/L	9.0–22.0 pmol/L
The blood film is reported as a dimorphic film with remnants of nuclear material (Howell–Jolly bodies) in some of the red blood cells.			

Differentials

- Coeliac disease
- Small intestinal bacterial overgrowth
- IBS

Coellac Disease

Insensitivity to gluten

Signs and symptoms

Chronic/intermittent steatorrhea
Failure to thrive
Unexplained GI symptoms

Macrocytic anaemia (folate/B12 deficiency)

Complications

Anaemia
Hyposplenism (=> Howell-Jolly bodies)
Osteoporosis
Lactose intolerance
T cell lymphoma

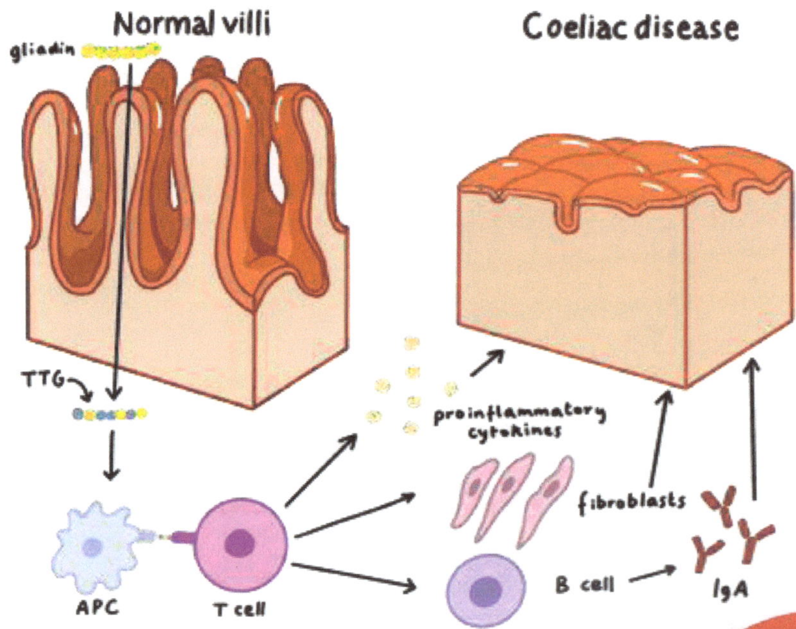

Coeliac disease Ix

Bedside: Observations

Bloods: FBC

Imaging: Small bowel endoscopy, small bowel histology

Special tests: tTG & IgA

Coeliac Disease Mx

Conservative

Gluten free diet

Medical

Vitamin and mineral supplementation

Surgical Nil

Note on management framework:
For acute scenarios, acute & definitive
For chronic/long term mx: Conservative, Medical, Surgical

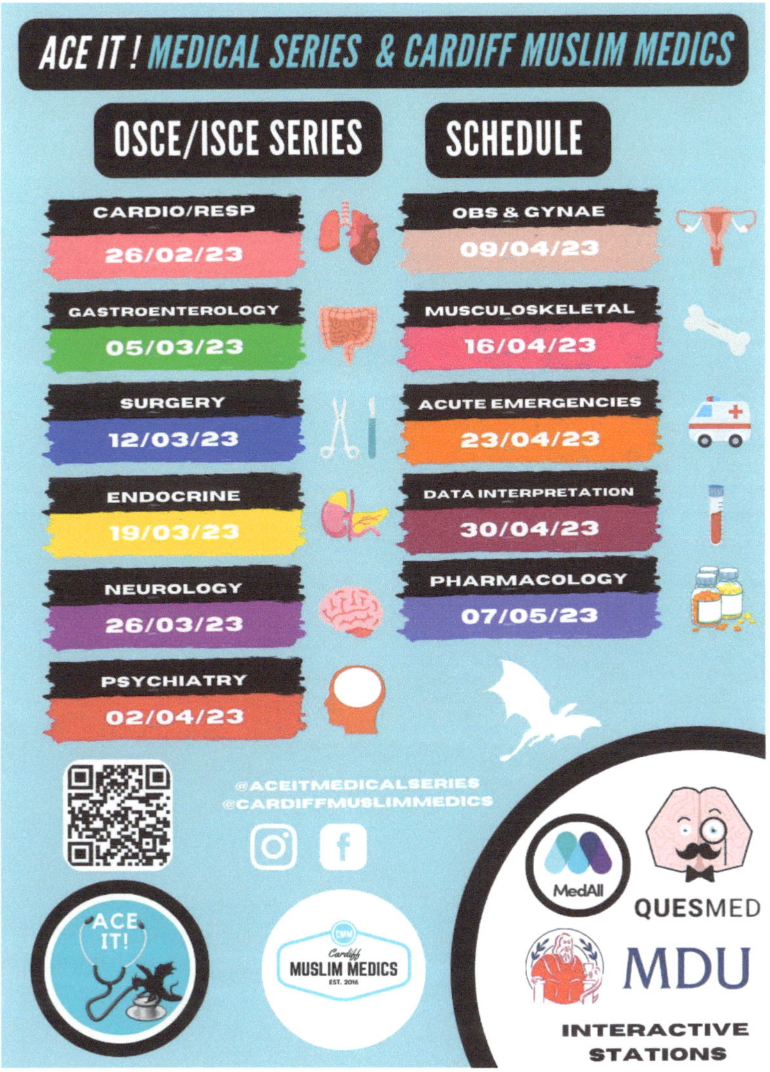

THANK YOU FOR LISTENING! 😊

ANY QUESTIONS?

Cardiff

MUSLIM MEDICS

EST. 2016

FEEDBACK FORM FOR SLIDES

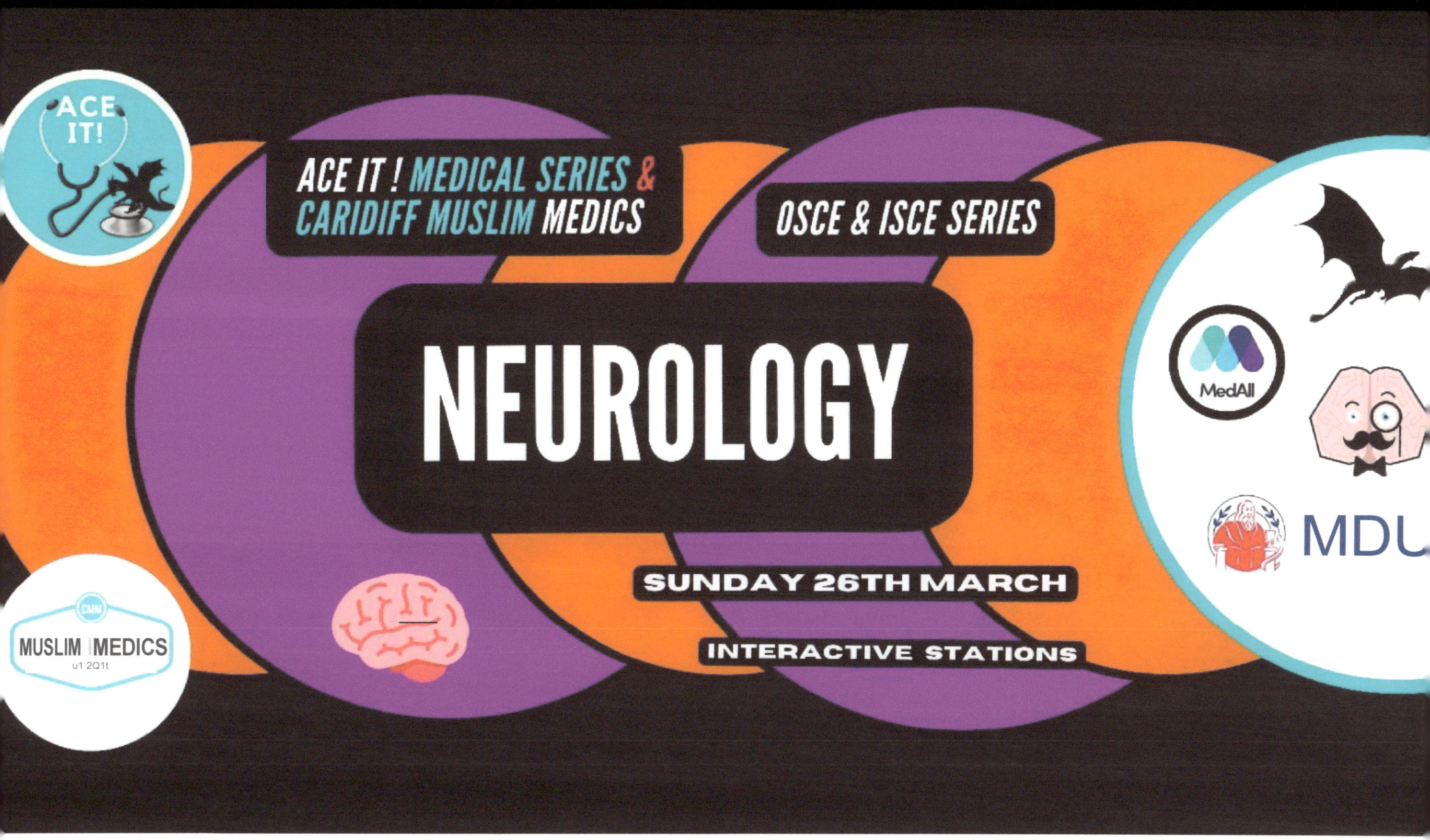
ACE IT!
ACE IT ! MEDICAL SERIES &
CARIDIFF MUSLIM MEDICS
OSCE & ISCE SERIES
NEUROLOGY
SUNDAY 26TH MARCH
INTERACTIVE STATIONS
MedAll
MDU
MUSLIM MEDICS

Yasmina Abdelrazik
FY1 Doctor

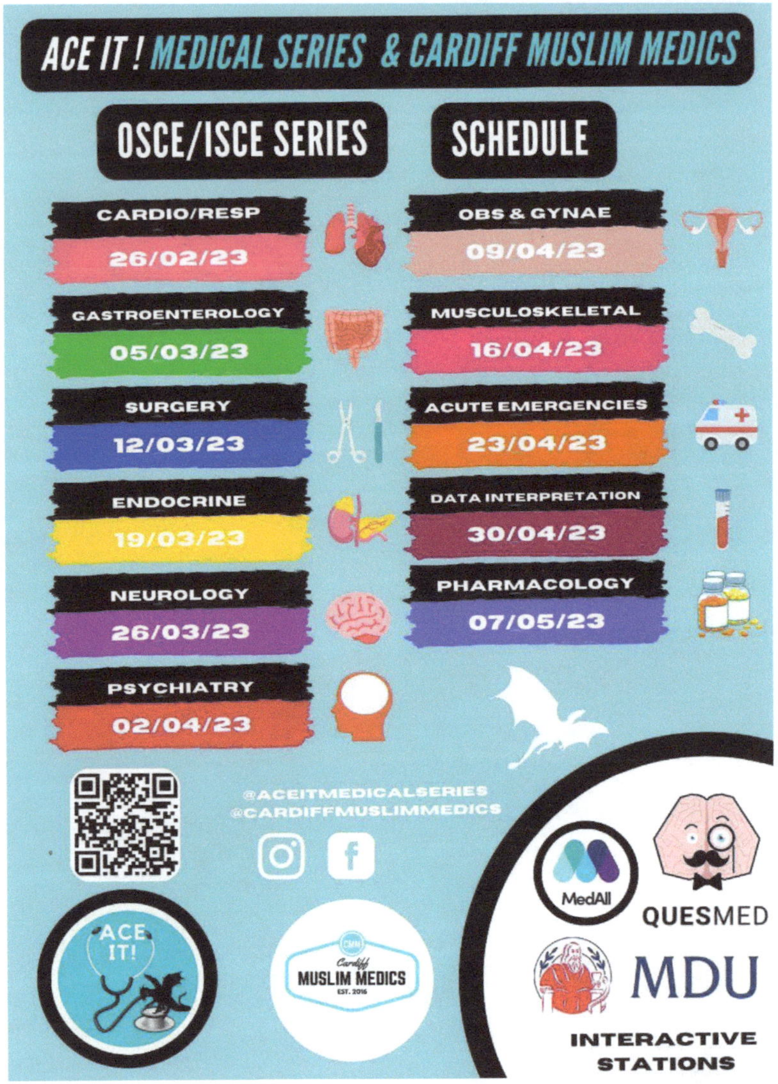

CMM
Cardiff
MUSLIM MEDICS
EST. 2016

Disclaimer

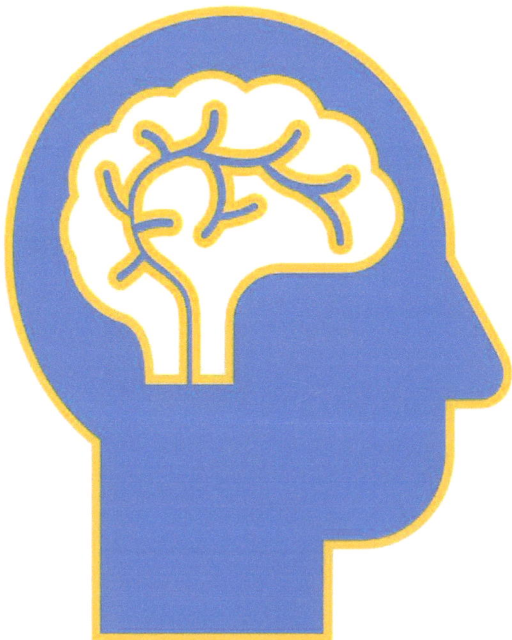

This is not an exhaustive list of everything you need to know. We have covered the main points to not forgot. Please refer to official guidelines for further information required.

Starter Pack: The history

What to NOT to Forget:

General neurological review
- Trauma
- Fits/ falls
- dizziness
- LOC
- Weakness
- Altered sensation

Back pain
- Incontinence
- Saddle anesthesia
- Neurological deficit
- Weight loss, fever, night sweats, cancer history, trauma

Headache Red flag symptoms
- Meningitis: fever, stiffness, photophobia, rash
- Sudden occipital headache
- New neurological deficit
- Temporal arteritis : visual problems, jaw claudication, scalp tenderness
- Glaucoma: visual problems, red eyes, halos
- Disturbs sleep
- Trauma
- Pregnancy
- Raised ICP

Raised ICP symptoms
- Headache worse in morning
- Positional- worse flat, straining
- Vomiting
- Reduced GCS
- Neurological deficit

Seizures/ Falls
- Check the cardiorespiratory system: chest pain, palpitations, SOB, cough

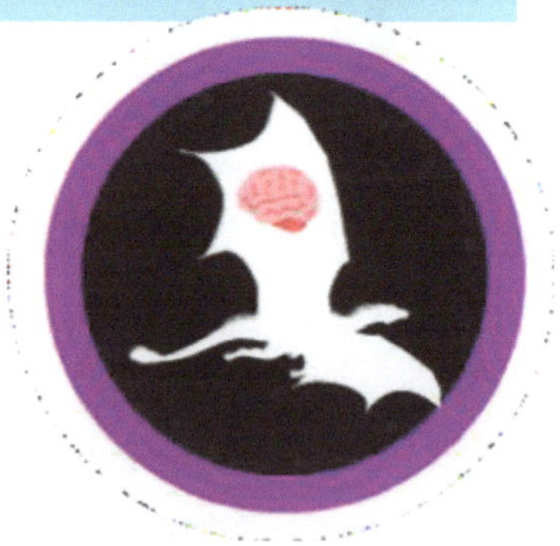

Starter Pack: Differentials

Vascular
Haemorrhage
Infarction

Infection
Meningitis, Encephalitis, Lyme disease, HIV, syphilis

Trauma+ Toxins
Alcohol
Drugs

Autoimmune
Diabetes Multiple sclerosis
Hyper/hypothyroidism
Sarcoidosis, every vasculitis

Metabolic
Encephalopath y Inherited conditions

Iatrogenic
Steroid myopathy
Radiotherapy
Drugs

Neoplastic + Nutritional
B12 defficiency
Thiamine defficiency

Congenital
Wilsons syndrome

Degenerative
Parkinson's
MND

Starter Pack: Investigations

Bedside	Full neurological exam including cranial nerves, vital signs, urine dip, BM
Bloods	FBC, U+Es, LFTs, CRP, Ca2+, B12, Folate, TFTs, HIV, Lyme disease, auto-antibody screen, coag, group + save/ cross match
Orifices	PR exam, swab
X-Ray	Imaging: Chest X-ray, CT, MRI
ECG	Routine, check for arrythmias
Special tests	Lumbar puncture, EMG, visual evoked potentials

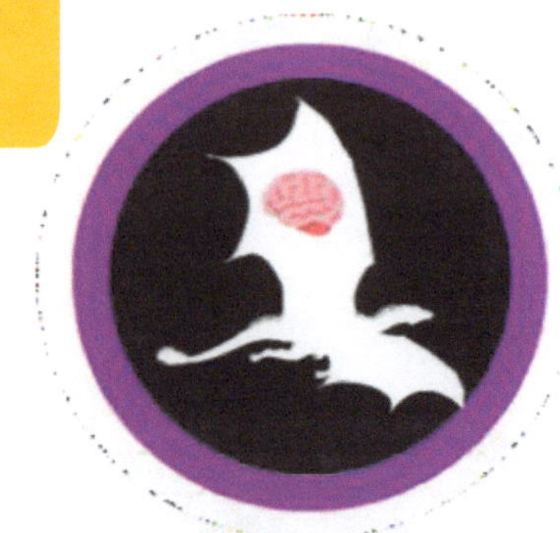

Starter Pack: Approach to Management

Can always say 'patient education + MDT approach'

1. CONSERVATIVE

Can always say 'full medication review'

2. MEDICAL

3. SURGICAL

Starter Pack: How to avoid red flags

DVLA□ almost everything in neuro

Say when something is a medical or surgical emergency

Say “I would also ask for senior review and input”

Station 1

Sara a 33-year-old woman presents to the emergency department with left leg heaviness and paresthesia

Differentials?

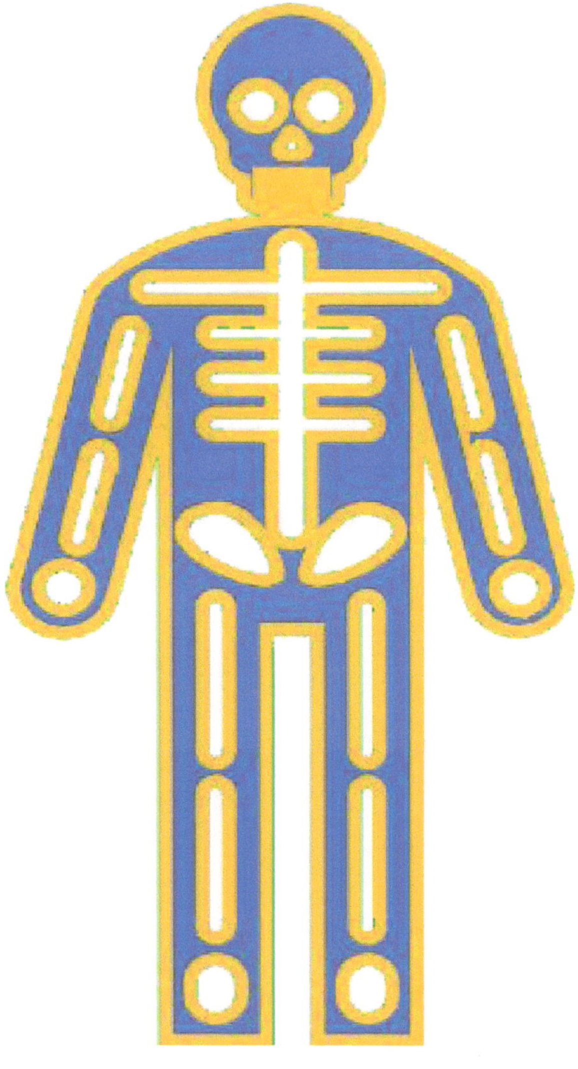

Differentials?

- TOP: MS
- MUST EXCLUDE: Stroke
- SOL
- B12 Deficiency
- Myelopathy
- GBS

How would you investigate this patient?

Bedside	Full neurological exam including cranial nerves, BM
Bloods	FBC, U+Es, LFTs, CRP, ESR,TFT's, Ca^{2+}, HIV, Lyme, syphilis
Orifices	N A
X-Ray	Imaging: MRI scan, chest X-ray (routine)
ECG	Routine A-E approach - exclude cardiac arrythmia (AF in particular)
Special tests	CSF analysis: oligoclonal bands not in serum, increased Ig G Visual evoked potential

Your MRI comes back:

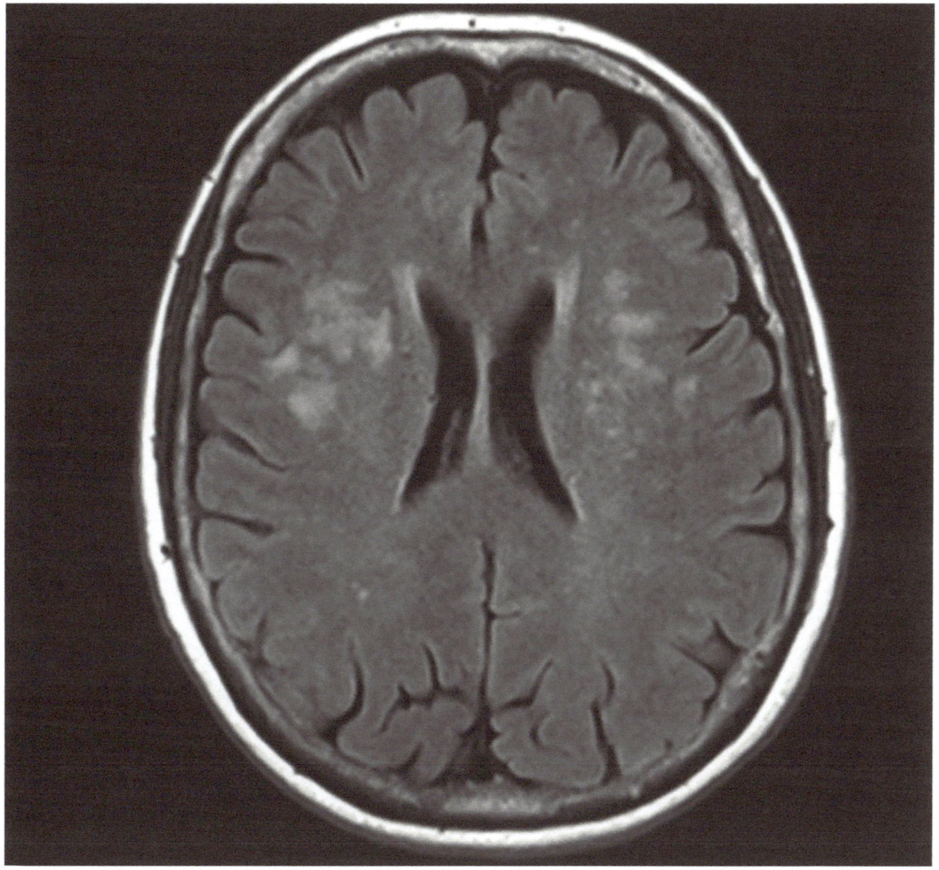

Image from:
https://dizziness-and-balance.com/disorders/central/pvm.htm

Your MRI comes back:

FIRST: check for correct patient details, date, time

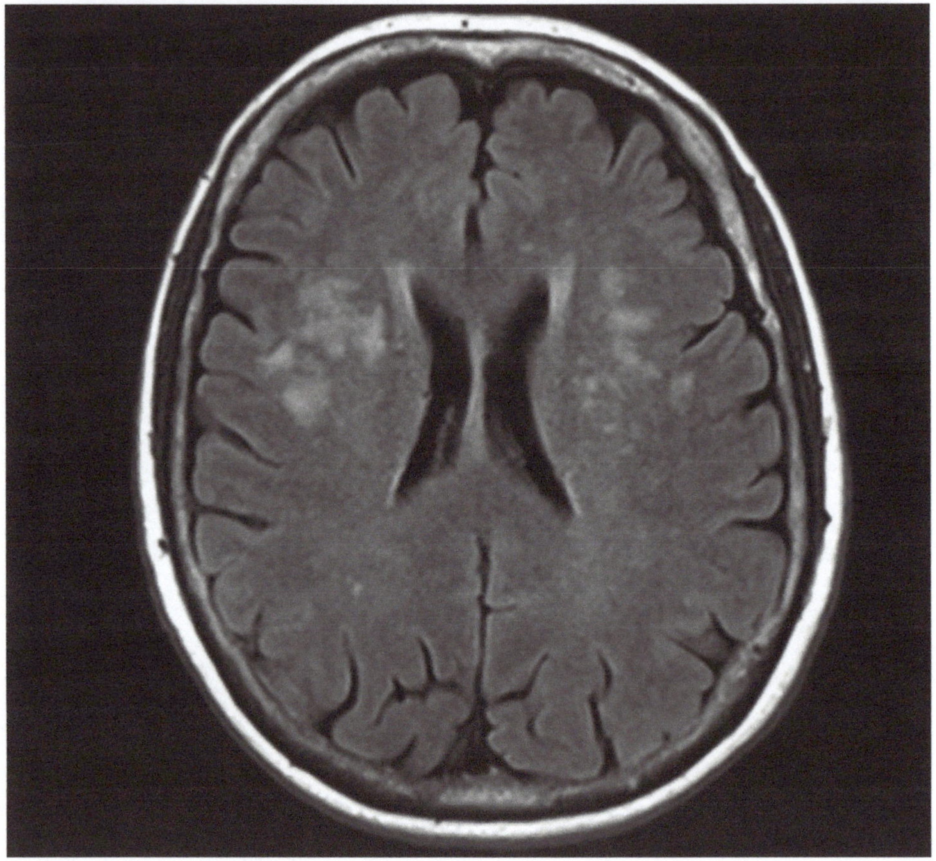

'This is a T1 weighted axial MRI scan of the head showing periventricular lesions indicative of MS'

Image from:
https://dizziness-and-balance.com/disorders/central/pvm.htm

How would you manage this patient?

MS Management

1. CONSERVATIVE

Refer to neurology
Specialist MDT
approach Patient
education
Psychosocial + Lifestyle: support groups, excersie,
smoking cessation
Inform DVLA

2. MEDICAL

Symptomatic treatment:
Spasticity- baclofen
Neuropathic pain- amitriptyline/
gabapentin Depression- SSRI
Urge incontinence- oxybutynin or
self-catheterisation Fatigue: amantadine,
physiotherapy or psychotherapy **Relapse
management:**
Acute relapse: methylprednisolone (+/- plasma
exchange) Disease modifying drugs- glatiramer
acetate, interferon beta
Biological therapy- natalizumab

Station 2

Ali, a 54-year-old man presents to the emergency department with right sided weakness.

Please take a focused history.

Before starting the station take 1 minute to think through all the possible differentials and how you are going to address them in the history…

Differentials

TOP: Stroke

SOL

Seizure - esp.Todd's pals

Sepsis,

Meningoencephalitis

History

PC **PMH**

Right sided weakness High cholesterol

HPCT2 Diabetes

Onset- 1.5 hours **DH**

No pain Simvastatin

Reduced sensation on R side Metformin

No headaches **FH**
No speech disturbance High blood pressure

No trauma to head **SH**

No neck stiffness Smoker
Didn't lose consciousness 1 glass of wine a

day Been feeling well **ICE**

No changes to visionAm I going to die?

O/E:

Both upper and lower L-sided weakness.

Power 3/5 on left, 5/5 on right.

Sensation intact.

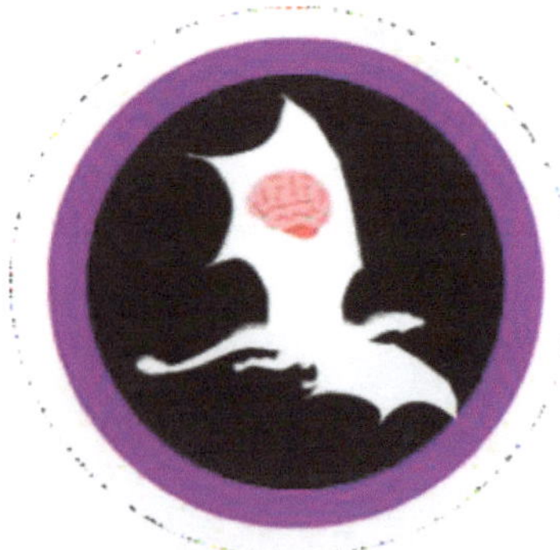

How would you investigate this patient?

Bedside	Full neurological exam including cranial nerves, BM, NIHSS, ROSIER
Bloods	FBC, U+Es, LFTs, CRP, ESR, Ca2+, Cholesterol, coag, group+ save/ crossmatch
Orifices	
X-Ray	Imaging: Urgent CT scan, diffusion weighted MRI scan (GOLD standard), chest X-ray (routine)
ECG	Routine A-E approach - exclude cardiac arrythmia (AF in particular)
Special tests	

CT Scan

Patient Name: Ali Hassan Patient

DOB: 07/01/1968

Hospital Number: 123456789

Date: 21/04/2022

Time: 17:05

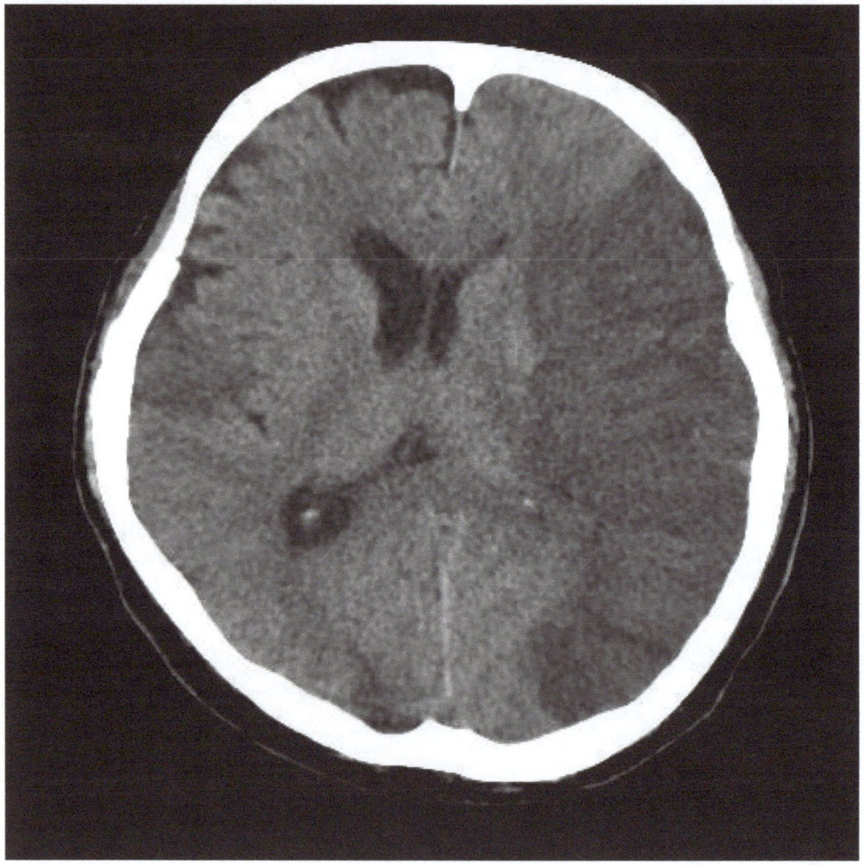

Image from: https://emedicine.medscape.com/article/338385-overview

CT Scan

Patient Name: Ali Hassan Patient
DOB: 07/01/1968
Hospital Number: 123456789
Date: 21/04/2022
Time: 17:05

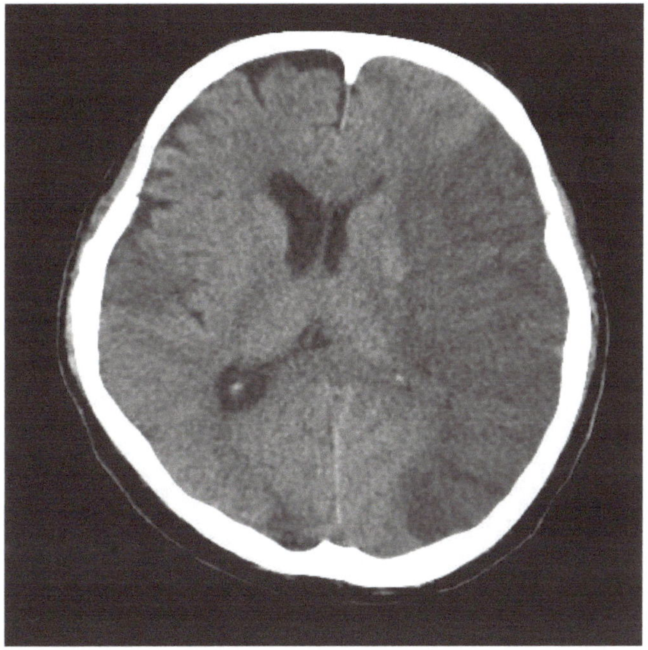

'This is an axial non-contrast CT scan of the Head showing hypodensity in the left frontal, parietal and temporal lobe. There is rightwad midline shift and sulcal effacement. This is indicative of left MCA infarct.'

Image from:
https://emedicine.medscape.com/article/338385-overview

How would you manage this patient?

Stroke Management

1. CONSERVATIVE	Imaging within 1 hour Supportive care- regular monitoring of vital signs VTE prophylaxis- stockings
2. MEDICAL	Aspirin 300mg (continued for 2 two weeks) If present within <4.5 hours □ thrombolysis e.g. Alteplase If present >24 hours only STAT aspirin 300mg
3. SURGICAL	Consider thrombectomy within 6 hours of symptom onset or up to 24 hours from onset if salvageable brain tissue
4. LONG TERM	Conservative: lifestyle advice, inform DVLA, smoking cessation, MDT approach: stroke nurse, SALT, nutrition, physio, OT Medical: - Clopidogrel or Aspirin + dipyridamole - Simvastatin Surgical: Carotid endarterectomy or stenting

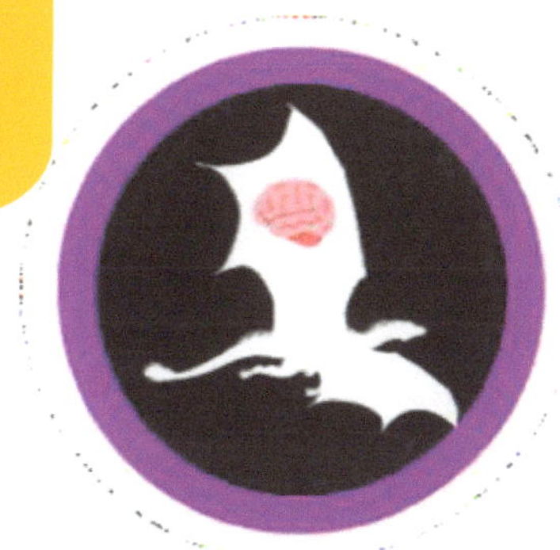

What if the symptoms had resolved?

TIA Management

1. CONSERVATIVE

A□ E exam, ABCD2 score + senior review
TIA >7 days □ specialist assessment within 7 days TIA <7 days □ urgent assessment within 24 hours Supportive care- regular monitoring of vital signs

2. MEDICAL

Aspirin 300mg (unless contraindicated)
Start statin 80mg
Anticoagulate if AF

3. SURGICAL

Carotid endarterectomy or stenting if >70% stenosis*

4. LONG TERM

Conservative: lifestyle advice, smoking cessation, MDT approach, inform DVLA
Medical:
- Clopidogrel 75 mg lifelong (2nd line: Aspirin 75mg)

Station 3

Fatima a 42-year-old presents to the emergency department with the ‘worst headache ever’.

Headache differentials?

Differential

- MUST EXCLUDE: subarachnoid haemorrhage
- MUST EXCLUDE:
- MUST EXCLUDE:
- MUST EXCLUDE: Temporal
- Migraine
- Cluster Headache
- Trauma
- Sinusitis

How would you investigate this patient?

Bedside	Full neurological exam including cranial nerves, BM
Bloods	FBC, U+Es, LFTs, CRP, coag, group+ save/ cross match
Orifices	
X-Ray	Imaging: Urgent CT scan, chest X-ray (routine)
ECG	ST elevation may be seen
Special tests	LP: 12 hours post headache if CT negative Digital subtractional catheter angiography (gold standard)

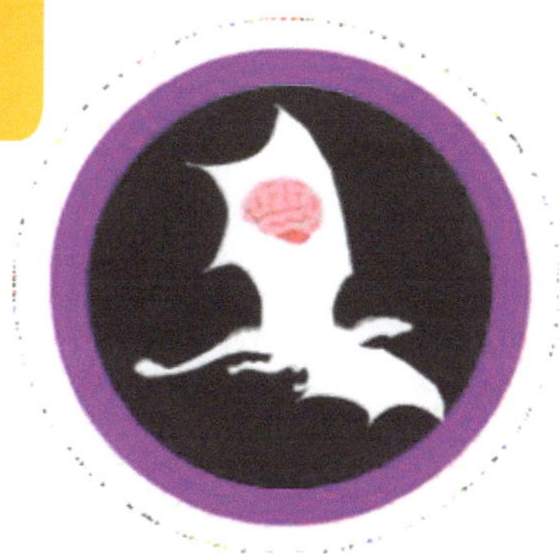

Your CT scan comes back...

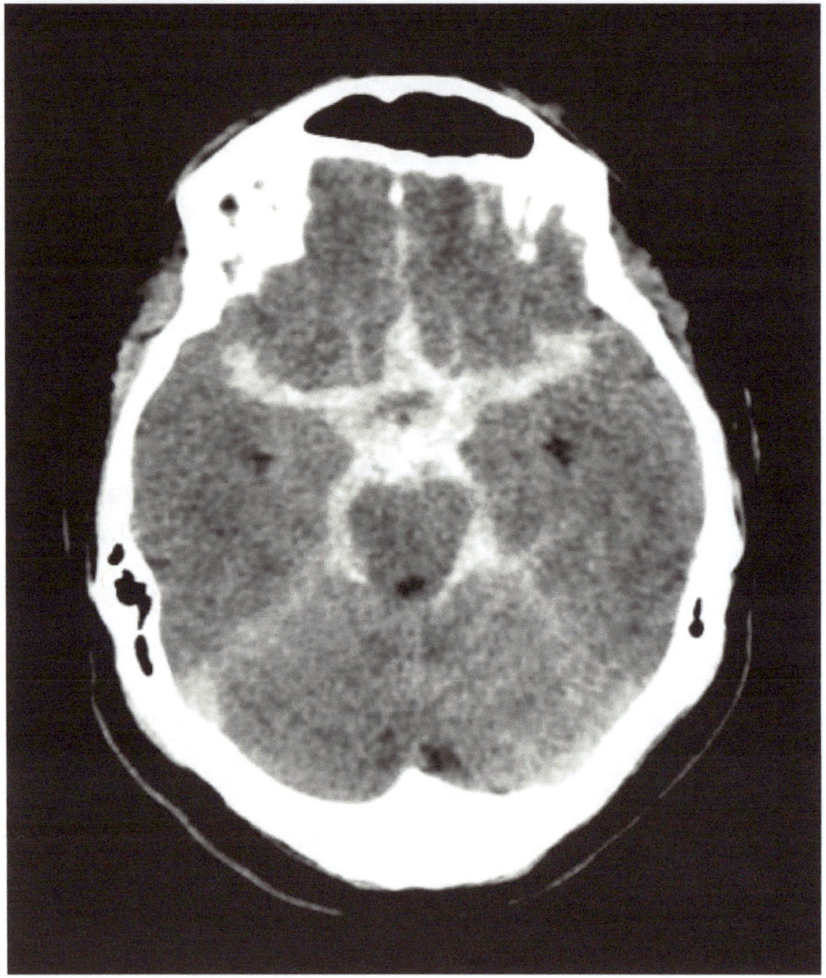

Image from:
https://radiopaedia.org/cases/subarachnoid-haemorrhage-4

Your CT scan comes back...

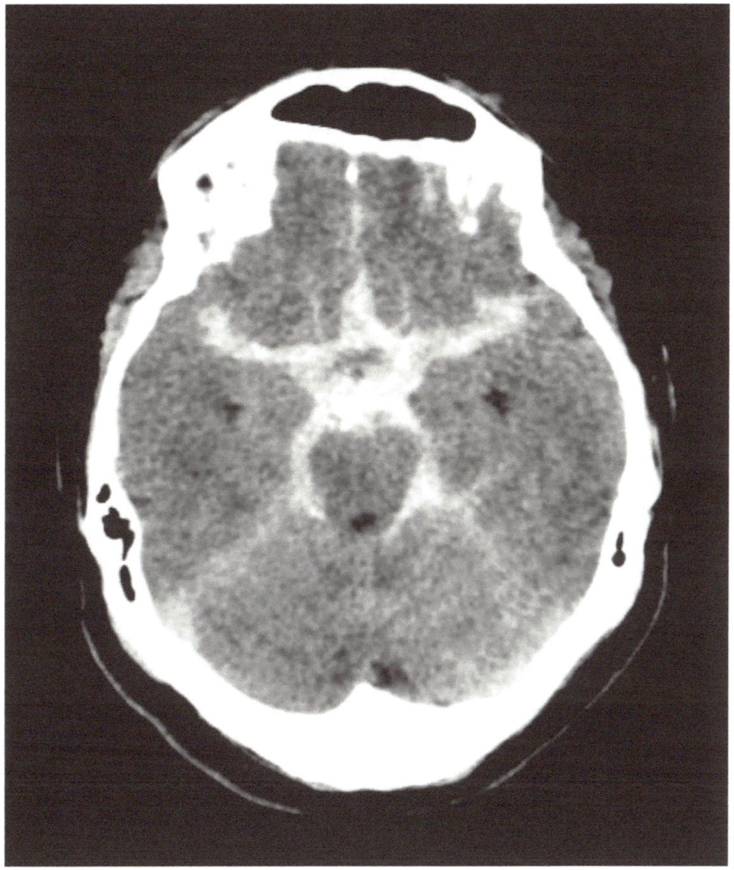

'This is a non-contrast axial CT scan of the head showing hyper density all basal cisterns, the bilateral sylvian fissures and inter-hemispheric fissure. This is consistent with a subarachnoid haemorrhage.'

Image from:
https://radiopaedia.org/cases/subarachnoid-haemorrhage-4

Your Lumbar Puncture comes back…

Opening pressure: Increased

Appearance: Yellow

RBC’s: Present

Xanthochromia: Present

How would you manage this patient?

Subarachnoid Haemorrhage Management

1. CONSERVATIVE	ABCDE + senior review + urgent referral to neurosurgery Bedrest + BP control Supportive care- regular monitoring of vital signs VTE thromboprophylaxis (TED stockings)
2. MEDICAL	Nimodipine (21 day course to stop vasospasm)
3. SURGICAL	Coil or craniotomy and clipping Hydrocephalus- external ventricular drain
4. LONG TERM	Conservative: lifestyle advice, smoking cessation, MDT approach: stroke nurse, physio, OT, inform DVLA Medical: address comorbidities

Station 4

Harry a 61-year-old presents to the GP with loss of sensation in his hands and feet.

Sensory neuropathy differentials?

Differentials

Diabetic neuropathy

Alcoholism

Drugs (amiodarone, isoniazid, nitrofurantoin)

B12/ thiamine defficiency

Vasculitis

How would you investigate this patient?

Bedside	Full peripheral vascular examination, ABPI, BM
Bloods	FBC, U+Es, LFTs, CRP, ESR, B12, folate,TFT's, autoantibody screen, cholesterol
Orifices	
X-Ray	
ECG	
Special tests	Consider nerve conduction studies

A focused history reveals that this patient is a type 2 diabetic. His HBA1c is 52mmol/mol.

How would you manage this patient?

Diabetic Neuropathy Management

1. CONSERVATIVE

Patient education□ better diabetic control Lifestyle advice, inform DVLA
MDT approach- diabetes nurse, dietician, pain management
Team

2. MEDICAL

1) Review medications for diabetes as per guidelines
2) Symptom control:
   - Pain: amitriptyline, gabapentin, duloxetine
   - Gastroparesis: metoclopramide
   - GORD: PPIs
   - Depression: SSRI

Station 5

Katy a 15-year-old girl is bought into the emergency department by her mother after having an ‘odd’ fall.

Differentials of a fall?

Differentials

Seizure

Arrhythmia

Drugs (overdose or toxicity)

Vasovagal syncope

Mechanical fall

Fits/ Falls: The History

Say you would like a collateral history as well!

History of presenting complaint section

BEFORE

-When?
-Where?
- What?
-Warning signs? Vision?
-Dizziness, chest pain, palpitations?

DURING

- LOC?
- Incontinence? Tongue biting?
- any injuries?
- What part of the body had first contact with the floor?
- Length?

AFTER

- Memory?
- Confusion?
- Tiredness after?
- Any muscle weakness/ altered sensation/ speech difficulty
- Who took you to the hospital?

Do a full **med review** in DH

Back to the patient...

The history reveals

- Loss of consciousness, no memory
- 2 minutes of jerking movements
- Still tired for 3 hours after
- No drug/ alcohol use
- First time to experience an event like this
- DH: oral contraceptive pill

Causes of seizures
Epilepsy (unidentified cause)
Epilepsy post trauma, stroke, SOL
Alcohol, drugs + withdrawal
Psychogenic non-epileptic seizures
Pre-eclampsia
Metabolic disturbances

How would you investigate this patient?

Bedside	Vital signs, full neurological examination, lying standing, BP, BM, pregnancy test
Bloods	FBC, U+E's, LFT's, bone profile, toxicology screen, prolactin+ CK
Orifices	
X-Ray	Imaging: chest X-ray, CT head
ECG	Bradycardia, arrythmia
Special tests	Electroencephalogram (eleptiform activity)

Epilepsy Management

Generalised tonic colonic seizure:

1. CONSERVATIVE	Refer to first seizure clinic Patient education Inform DVLA + do NOT drive
2. MEDICAL	Lamotrigine (sodium valproate and carbamazepine contraindicated)
3. SURGICAL	Only if structural abnormality

Generalised tonic colonic seizure	Focal seizure	Absence seizure
1st line: sodium valproate 2nd line: lamotrigine or carbamazepine	1st line: lamotrigine or carbamazepine 2nd line: sodium valproate or levetiracetam	1st line: sodium valproate or ethosuximide NB: Avoid Carbamazepine

Station 6

Henry a 72-year-old man presents to the GP with a tremor, stiffness and difficulty walking.

Differentials

- Parkinson’s disease
- Parkinson’s dementia
- Drug-induced Parkinsonism
- Parkinson’s plus syndromes

How would you investigate this patient?

Refer to

Bedside	Full neurological exam, lying/ standing blood pressure, urine dip
Bloods	FBC, U+E's, LFT's,TFTs
Orifices	
X-Ray	Imaging: if diagnostic uncertainty □ single photon emission computed tomography (SPECT).
ECG	Routine (falls assessment)
Special tests	

History + Examination...

Characteristicall
y asymmetrical!

Motor Symptoms:

- Pill rolling **tremor**
- Cogwheel **rigidity**
- **Bradykinesia**
- Shuffling gait
- Mask like face
- Micrographic
- Microphonia

Non-motor symptoms

-**Neuropsychiatric problems:** depression, anxiety, apathy, hallucinations, impulse control disorder

-**Autonomic dysfunction:** dysphagia, constipation, urgency, incontinence, orthostatic hypotension, sexual dysfunction

- **Sleep disorders:** insomnia
- **Sensory disorders:** hyposmia, pain, paresthesia

To my knowledge.. Cardiff have not asked for a Parkinson's examination. It is usually an upper/lower motor neuron exam. But you may be asked about Parkinson's features in the questions.

Parkinson's Disease Management

1. CONSERVATIVE

Refer to PD specialist
MDT approach: specialist nurse, physio, OT, SALT, counselling Patient education
Inform DVLA

2. MEDICAL

1st line: Levodopa + dopa-decarboxylase inhibitor e.g. carbidopa (prevents peripheral conversion)
2nd line: Dopamine agonist e.g. bromocriptine or MOA-B inhibitors e.g. selegiline
3rd line: COMT inhibitors e.g. entacapone

3. SURGICAL

Deep brain stimulation for refractory symptoms

If you elicit signs in your neuro exam: back to the basics:

1) Break it down into UMN or LMN

UMN lesion	LMN lesion
Increased tone	decreased tone
Spasticity	Wasting and fasciculation
Hyperreflexia	Hyporeflexia
Weakness	Weakness

2) Is is bilateral or Unilateral

Bilateral UMN	Unilateral
MS	Intracranial: MS, CVA, SOL
Myelopathy	Brainstem: MS
MND	Spinal cord: MS,Trauma, SOL, abscess

If you elicit signs in your neuro exam: back to the basics:

3) for LMN divide it up into Bi/unilateral + whether sensation is intact or not

Bilateral LMN + altered sensation	Unilateral LMN
Diabetes mellitus	Radiculopathy (dermatomal sensory loss)
Metabolic: B12/ thiamine defficiency	Plexopathy (vast dermatomal sensory loss)
Infections: herpes zoster, HIV, Lyme, Syphilis	Nerve palsy
Toxins: alcohol, drugs e.g. amiodarone	
Inherited: CMT	
Bilateral LMN: intact sensation	
Guillain Barre syndrome	
Lambert Eaton syndrome	
Lead poising	

Finally: Spot diagnosis

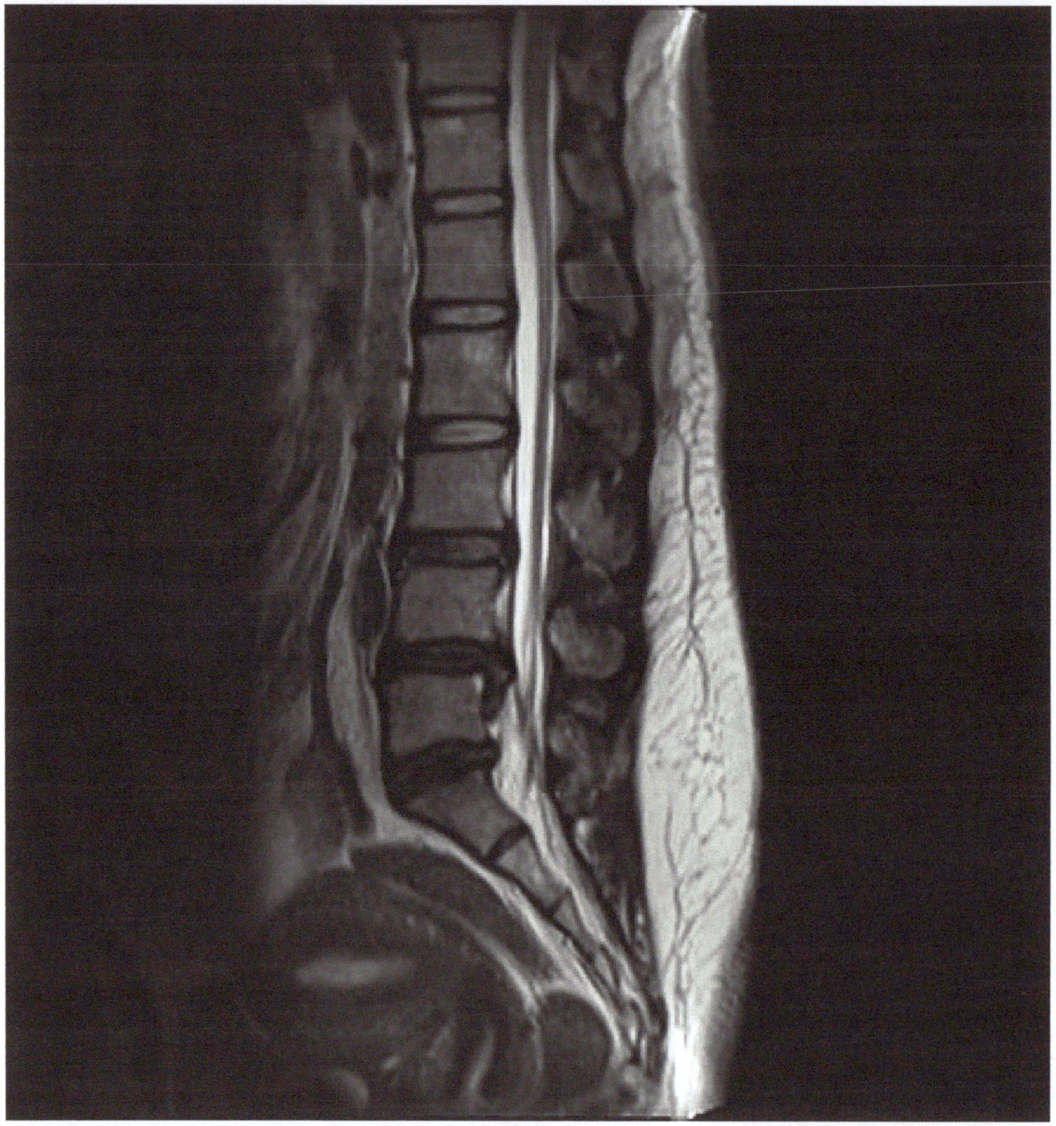

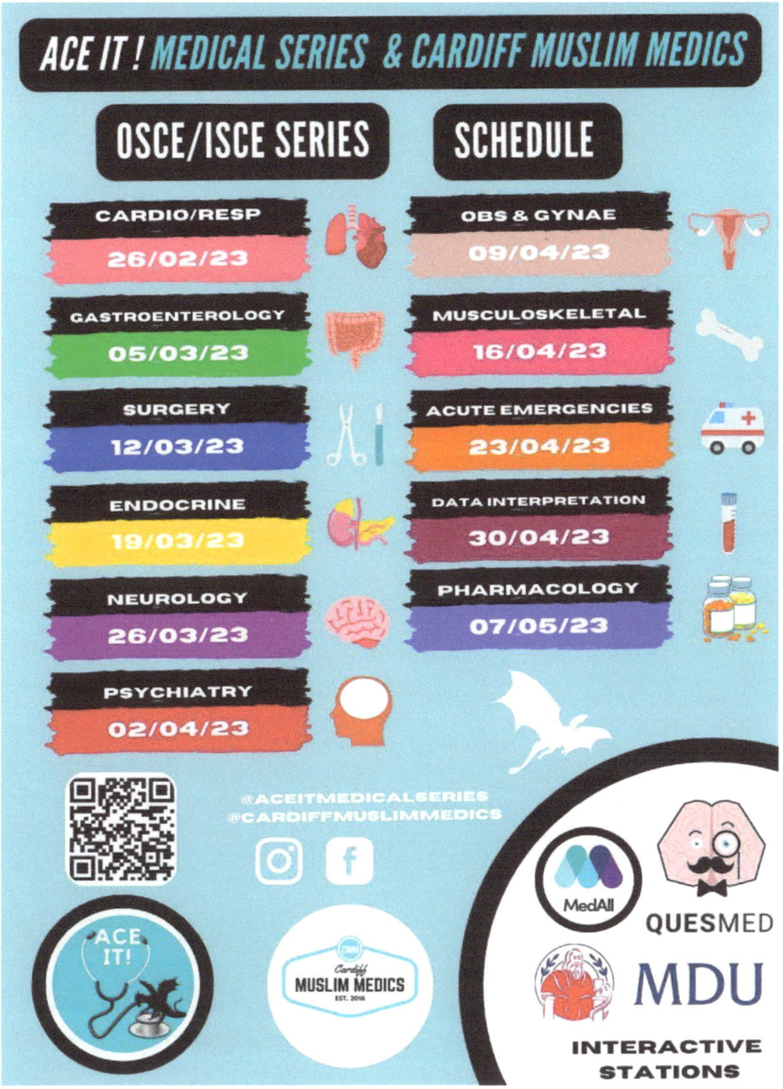

THANK YOU FOR LISTENING! 😊
ANY QUESTIONS?

Feeback form for slides

Examination Stations

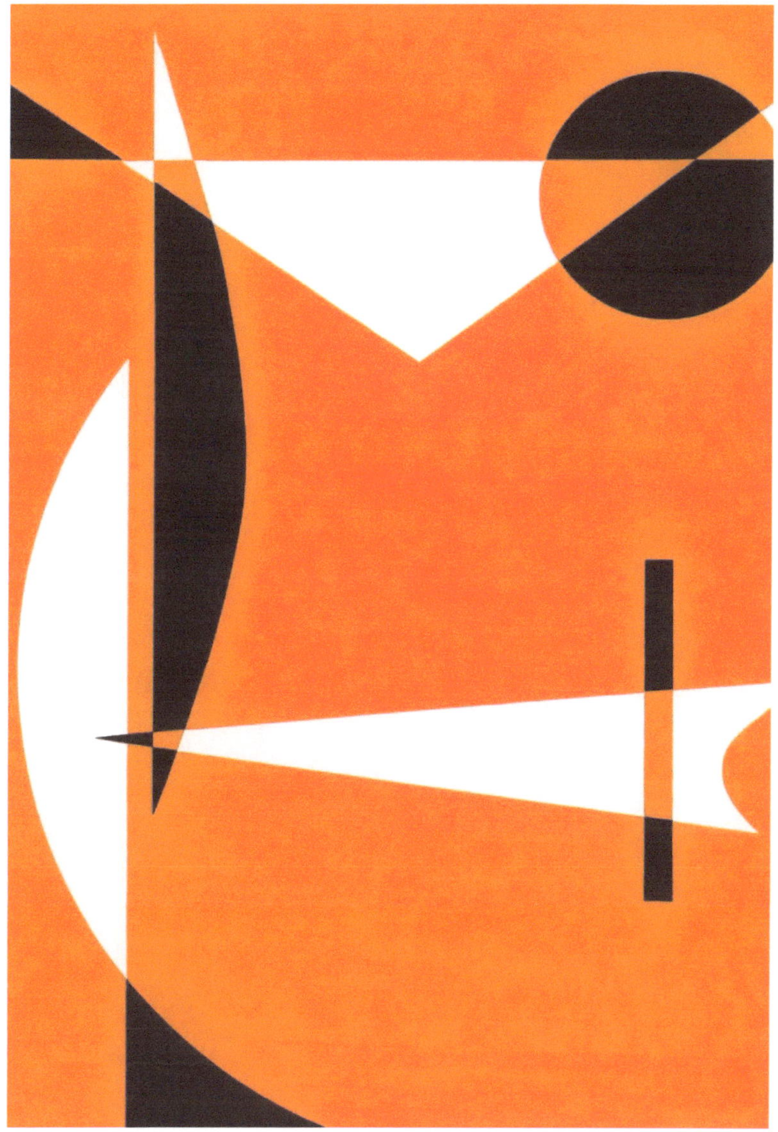

Eye exam

Introduction

- Wash hands, don PPE
- Introduce yourself, confirm patient identity
- Explain the procedure and gain consent
- Ask about pain or discomfort

Visual Acuity

- Distance vision: Snellen chart at 6 meters
  - Test each eye separately (with glasses if worn)
  - Record as 6/x (e.g., 6/6, 6/12)
  - If unable to read top line: move closer, then test CF, HM, PL
- Near vision: Use a near vision chart or printed text
- Pinhole test: If reduced acuity, test with pinhole to assess for refractive error

Visual Fields

- Confrontation method:
  - Sit opposite patient
  - Test each quadrant in both eyes
  - Compare with your own visual field
- Formal testing: Mention automated perimetry if relevant

Pupilary Reflex

- Size and symmetry
- Direct and consensual light reflex
- Swinging flashlight test: Check for RAPD
- Accommodation reflex: Focus on distant then near object

External Inspection:

- Eyebrows and eyelids: Ptosis, swelling, lesions
- Lacrimal apparatus: Swelling, discharge
- Conjunctiva and sclera: Redness, jaundice, injection
- Cornea and iris: Clarity, shape, scars

Eye exam

Eye movements:	Ask patient to follow your finger in an "H" pattern	Look for: • Nystagmus • Diplopia • Movement restriction	Ask about double vision or pain on movement	
Fundoscopy:	Red reflex: Present or absent	Optic disc: Color, margins, cup-to-disc ratio	Retinal vessels: Arteriovenous ratio, hemorrhages	Macula: Use direct gaze, assess foveal reflex
Colour Vision:	Use Ishihara plates	Test each eye separately	Note any color blindness or red-green defects	
Intraocular Pressure:	Mention tonometry (Goldmann or non-contact)	Normal range: 10–21 mmHg		
Additional Tests:	Amsler grid: Macular function	Cover test: Detect strabismus	Slit lamp: For anterior segment exam (if available)	Fluorescein staining: Detect corneal abrasions or ulcers

Visual Acuity:

Preparation

Ensure adequate lighting and a quiet environment.

Ask if the patient wears corrective lense test with and without them.

Use a Snellen chart at 6 meters (or 3 meters if space is limited)

Distance Vision (Snellen Chart)

How to Perform:

Cover one eye (without pressing on it).

Ask the patient to read the smallest line they can see clearly.

Repeat for the other eye.

Recording Results:

Format: 6/x, where:

6 = distance from chart (in meters)

x = distance at which a normal eye can read that line

Example: 6/6 = normal vision; 6/12 = patient sees at 6m what a normal eye sees at 12m

Near Vision

Use a near vision chart or printed text (e.g., newspaper).

Hold at reading distance (~35 cm). Test each eye separately.

Useful for detecting presbyopia or hypermetropia.

Pinhole Test

Use a pinhole occluder if acuity is reduced.

Improvement suggests refractive error (e.g., myopia, hyperopia).

No improvement suggests pathology (e.g., cataract, macular disease).

Repeat for the other eye.

Recording Results:

Format: 6/x, where:

6 = distance from chart (in meters)

x = distance at which a normal eye can read that line

Example: 6/6 = normal vision; 6/12 = patient sees at 6m what a normal eye sees at 12m

Visual Acuity:

☐ **Preparation**

Ensure adequate lighting and a quiet environment.

Ask if the patient wears corrective lense test with and without them.

Use a Snellen chart at 6 meters (or 3 meters if space is limited)

Repeat for the other eye.

Recording Results:

Format: 6/x, where:

- 6 = distance from chart (in meters)
- x = distance at which a normal eye can read that line

Example: 6/6 = normal vision; 6/12 = patient sees at 6m what a normal eye sees at 12m

🔍 Distance Vision (Snellen Chart) How to Perform:

Cover one eye (without pressing on it).

Ask the patient to read the smallest line they can see clearly.

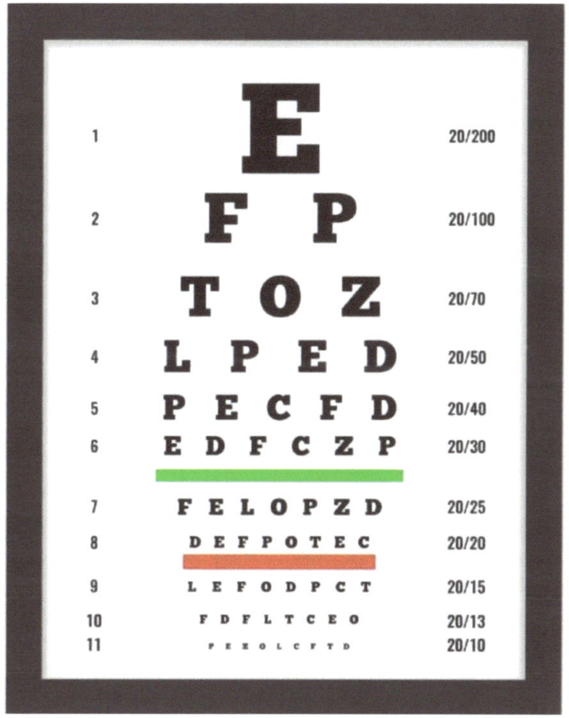

Visual Fields:

Preparation
Sit directly opposite the patient at eye level, about 1 meter apart.
Ask the patient to cover one eye (you cover the opposite eye).
Instruct them to look directly into your uncovered eye and not move their gaze.

Testing Each Quadrant
Extend your arms halfway between you and the patient.
Wiggle your fingers or use a small object (e.g., red-tipped pen).
Bring it in from the periphery toward the center in each of the four quadrants:

- Upper temporal
- Lower temporal
- Upper nasal
- Lower nasal

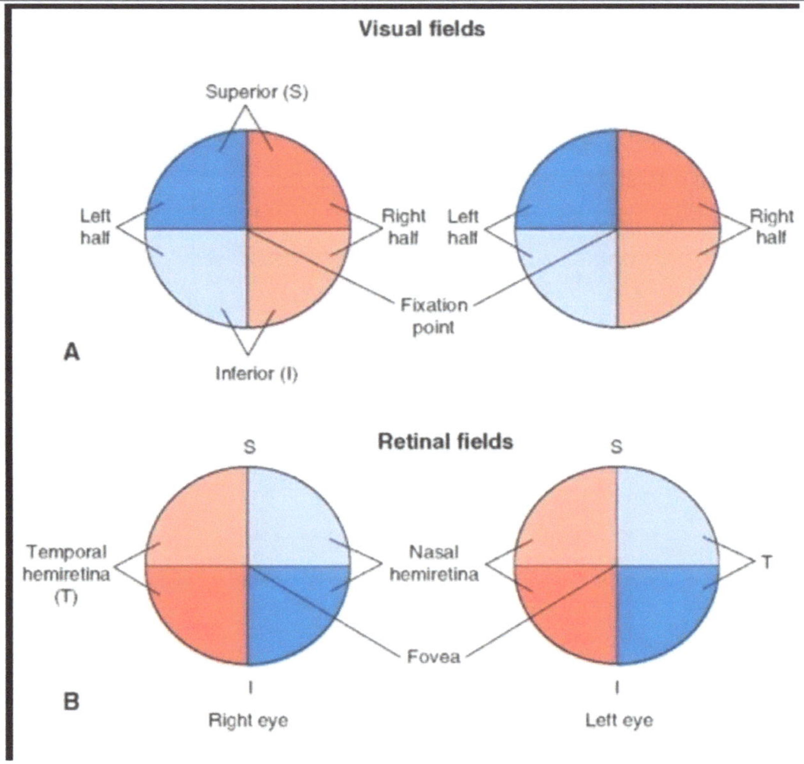

Visual Fields:

Technique:
Ask: "Tell me when you first see my fingers."
Compare their response to your own visual field.
Repeat for the other eye.

Note which eye was tested first. Record any deficits and their location.
Example: "Left eye: full visual fields. Right eye: upper temporal quadrant defect."
Always compare to your own field.
Be systematic: test all four quadrants. If abnormal, mention need for formal perimetry

□ Advanced Techniques (if needed) Red pin test: Use a red-tipped pin to detect subtle field defects.
Kinetic testing: Move the stimulus from periphery inward.
Static testing: Present stimulus at fixed points and ask if it's visible.

Visual fields

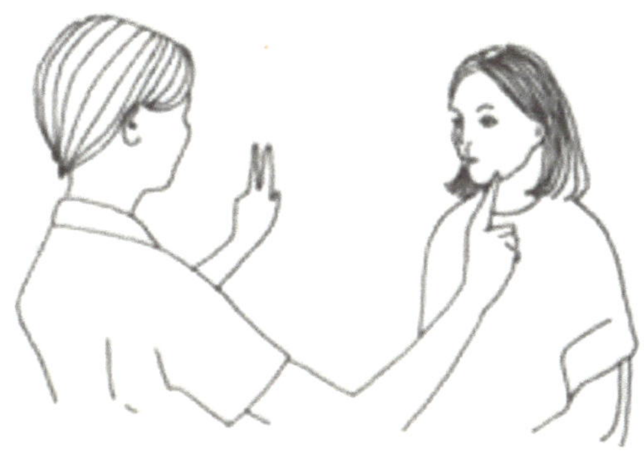

Visual Field Defects

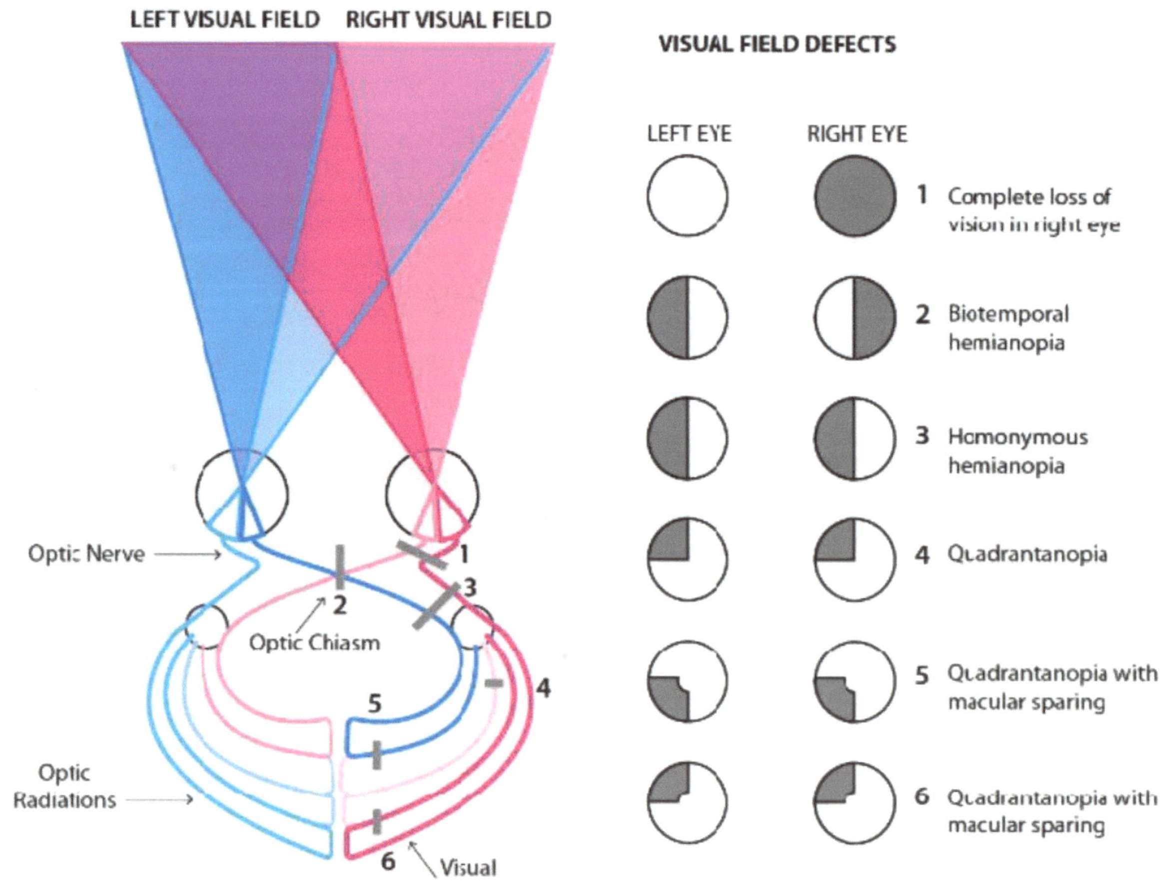

Shows visual field and possible visual impairments (Garrity, 2020).

Eye Movements

Set-Up
Position yourself at eye level with the patient.
Ask them to keep their head still and follow your finger with their eyes only.

Performing the H-TestMove your finger in an "H" shape to test:Horizontal gaze (lateral rectus – CN VI, medial rectus – CN III)Vertical gaze (superior/inferior rectus – CN III, superior oblique – CN IV)Pause at each extreme to check for nystagmus.

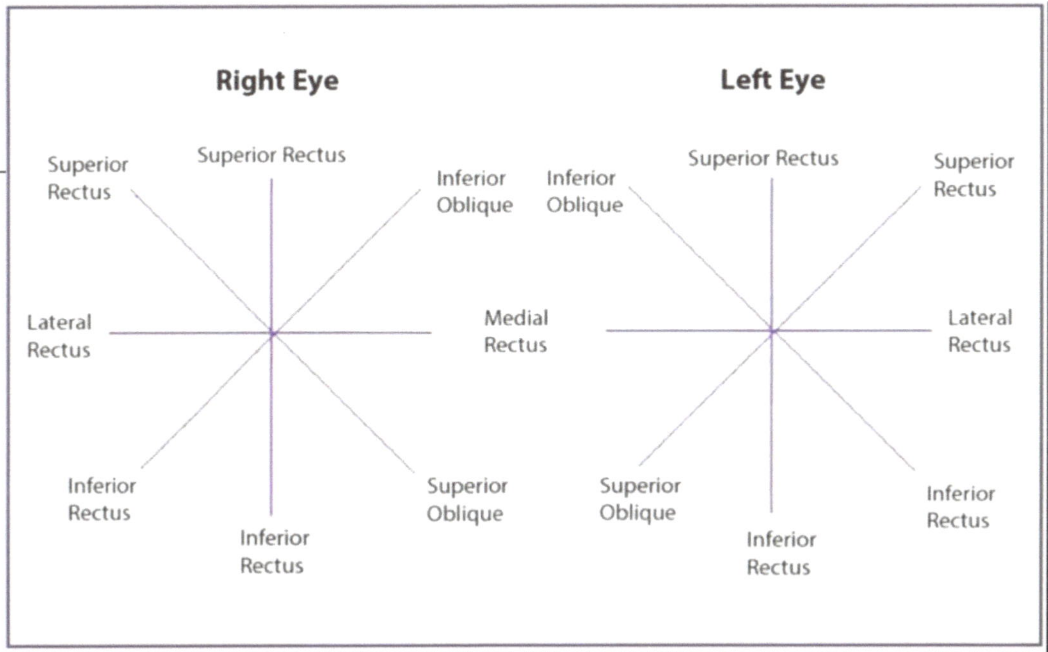

LR6 SO4, all the rest 3"
Lateral Rectus → CN VI (Abducens)
Superior Oblique → CN IV (Trochlear) All others → CN III (Oculomotor)

Eye Movements

- **Diplopia**: Ask if they see double at any point.
- **Ptosis or dilated pupil**: Think CN III palsy.
- **Down and out eye**: Classic CN III palsy.
- **Vertical diplopia worsens on downward gaze**: CN IV palsy.
- **Failure to abduct**: CN VI palsy

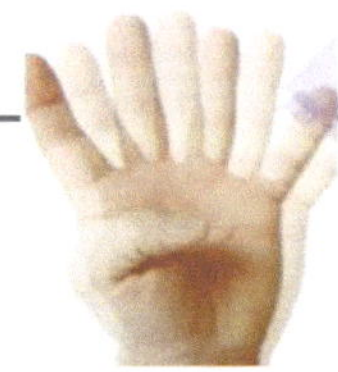

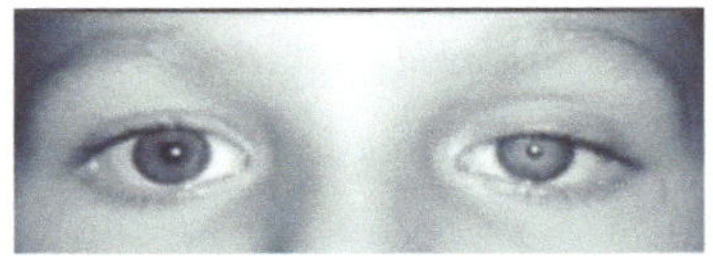

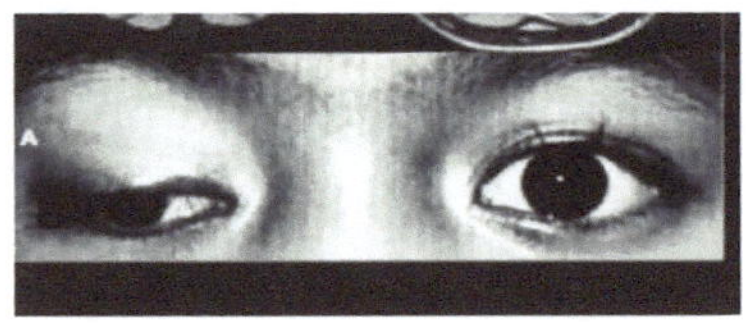

RIGHT 4th NERVE PALSY

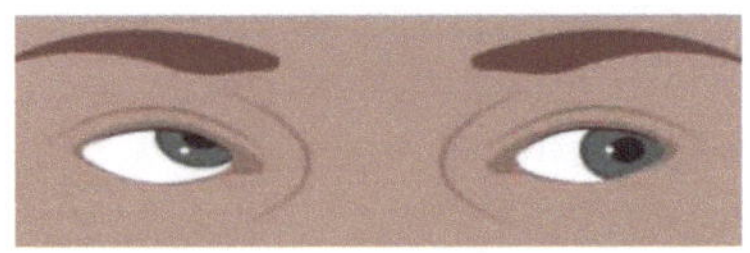

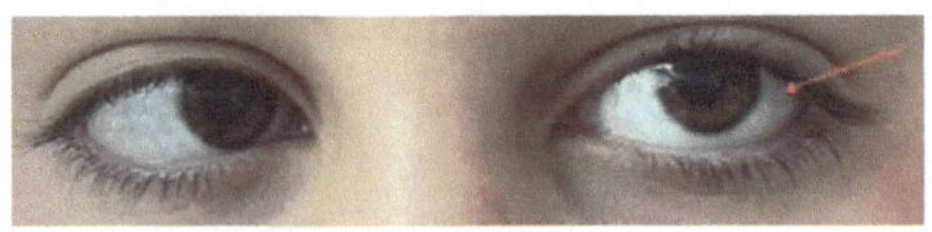

Pupillary Reflex

Types of Pupillary Reflexes

- Direct Light Reflex – Pupil constricts when light is shone directly into it.
- Consensual Light Reflex – Opposite pupil also constricts when light is shone into one eye.
- Accommodation Reflex – Pupils constrict when focusing from a distant object to a near one

Accommodation Reflex

Ask the patient to focus on a distant object.

Then ask them to shift gaze to a near object (e.g., your finger ~15 cm from their nose).

Observe pupillary constriction and convergence of the eyes.

Direct and Consensual Light Reflex. Use a pen torch. Shine light into one eye: Observe direct constriction. Observe consensual constriction in the opposite eye. Repeat for the other eye.

How it works?

Light enters one eye

The signal travels along the optic nerve (CN II)

It reaches the midbrain, specifically the pretectal nucleus

The response is sent out via the oculomotor nerve (CN III) Both pupils constrict — even if only one eye was stimulated Two key components:

Direct response: the pupil of the eye receiving the light constricts

Consensual response: the pupil of the opposite eye also constricts

Pupillary Reflex

- **Relative Afferent Pupillary Defect (RAPD)**:
  - Use the **Swinging Light Test**.
  - Shine light alternately between eyes.
  - Affected eye shows **dilation** when light is moved to it (instead of constriction).

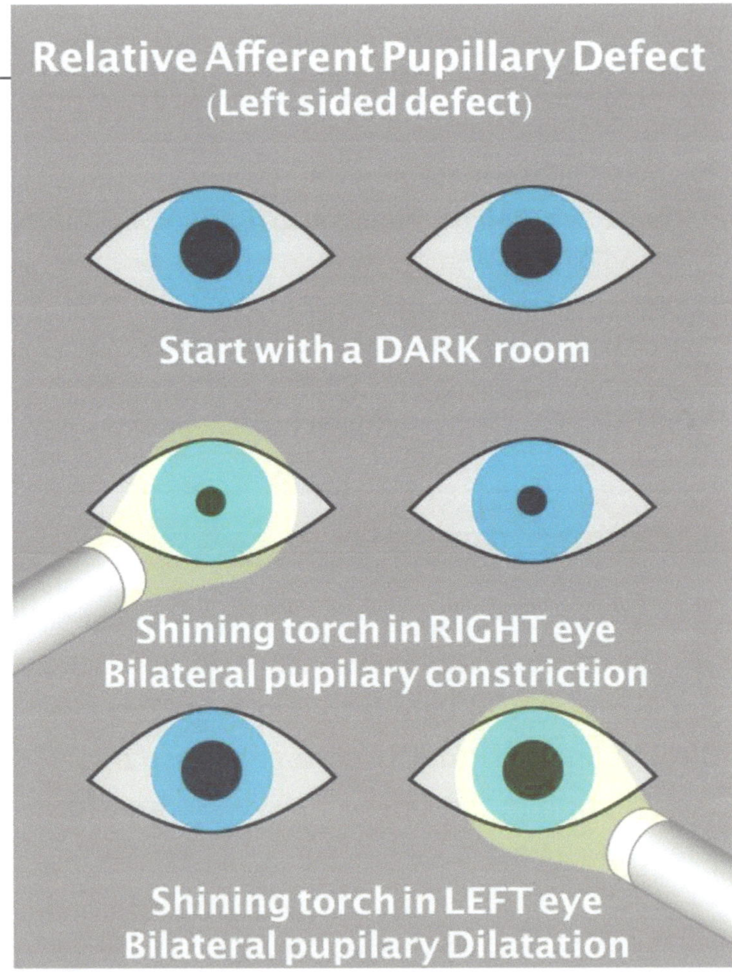

Pupillary Reflex

- **Argyll Robertson pupil**:
  - Pupils accommodate but don't react to light.
  - Seen in neurosyphilis.
- **Horner's syndrome**:
  - Miosis, ptosis, anhidrosis.
- **CN III palsy**:
  - Dilated pupil, ptosis, eye "down and out".

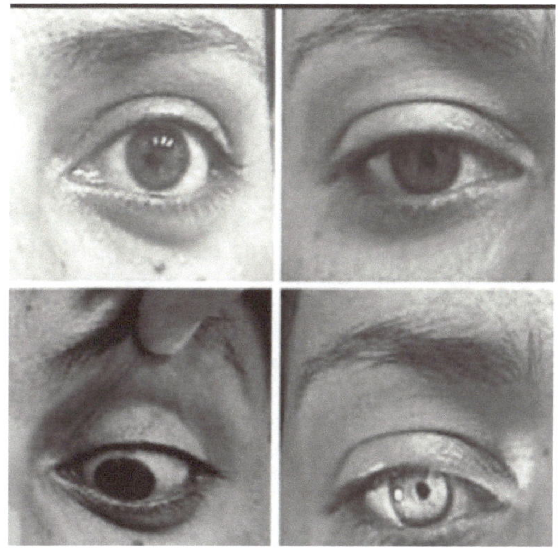

Fundoscopy

Equipment Used Ophthalmoscope:
Main tool with adjustable light and lenses.
Dilating Drops: Used to widen the pupil for better visualization.
Condensing Lens (for indirect): Enhances magnification and field of view.

Inspect:
Optic disc: Check for swelling, pallor, or cupping. Retinal vessels: Look for narrowing, hemorrhages, or exudates. Macula: Assess for degeneration or oedema. General retina: Detect lesions, tears, or detachment.

- **Positioning**:
  - Patient sits comfortably, looking straight ahead.
  - Examiner uses right eye and hand for patient's
  - right eye, and vice versa.

- **Examination**:
  - Darken the room to enhance pupil dilation.
  - Look for the **red reflex**—a glow from the retina.

  - Follow the red reflex to visualize the retina.

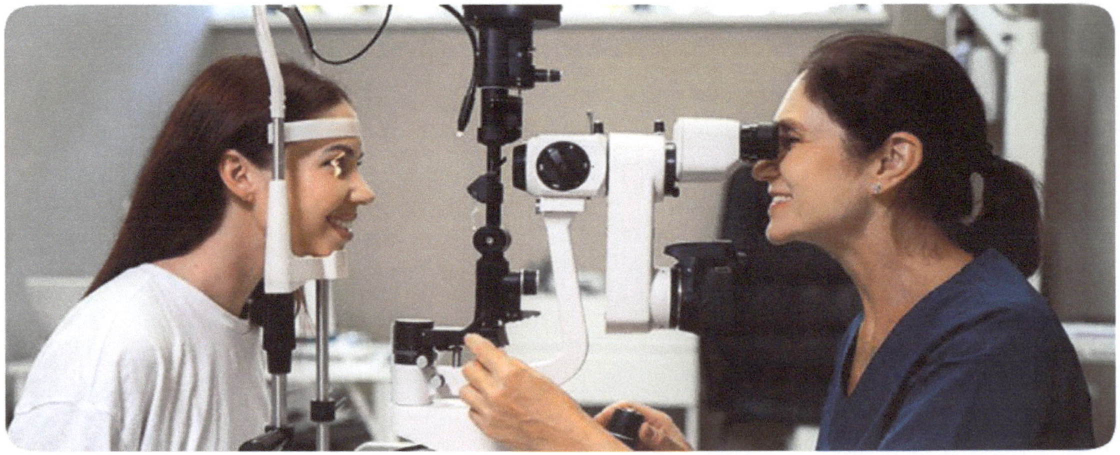

Fundoscopy

🔍 Retinal Vein occlusion
Cover one eye (without pressing on it).
Ask the patient to read the smallest line they can see clearly.

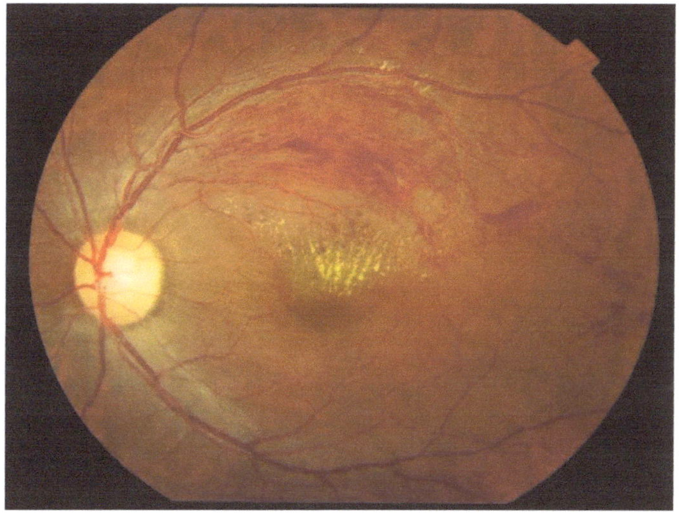

Pinhole Test
Use a pinhole occluder if acuity is reduced.
Improvement suggests refractive error (e.g., myopia, hyperopia).
No improvement suggests pathology (e.g., cataract, macular disease).

LR6 SO4, all the rest 3"
Lateral Rectus → CN VI (Abducens)
Superior Oblique → CN IV (Trochlear) All others → CN III (Oculomotor)

Cardiovascular Exam

General Inspection:
- Look for medical equipment (e.g. oxygen, ECG leads)
- Assess patient's appearance: breathlessness, cyanosis, pallor
- Check for signs around the bed (e.g. medications, mobility aids)

Hands and Arms
- Hands and Arms
- Inspect for clubbing, cyanosis, tar staining
- Palpate radial pulse (rate, rhythm)
- Check for collapsing pulse
- Assess capillary refill time
- Inspect for peripheral stigmata of endocarditis

Face and Neck
- Inspect eyes for pallor, xanthelasma
- Inspect mouth for central cyanosis, dental hygiene
- Assess jugular venous pressure (JVP)
- Palpate carotid pulse (one at a time)

Chest
- nspect for scars, deformities
- Palpate apex beat (5th intercostal space, midclavicular line)
- Assess for heaves and thrills

Auscultate Heart Sounds:
- Aortic (2nd right intercostal space)
- Pulmonary (2nd left intercostal space)
- Tricuspid (lower left sternal border)
- Mitral (apex)

Legs:
- Inspect for peripheral edem a
- Palpate pedal pulses
- Check for signs of deep vein thrombosis (DVT)

To complete the examination:
- Measure blood pressure
- Perform peripheral vascular exam if indicated
- Request ECG, chest X-ray, blood tests

Chest Exam: Murmurs

Murmurs Mnemonics
Use "MR PASS MVP" to remember systolic vs diastolic murmurs:
Systolic Murmurs:
MR: Mitral Regurgitation
PASS: Pulmonary and Aortic Stenosis Diastolic Murmurs:
MVP: Mitral and Tricuspid Stenosis
AR: Aortic Regurgitation
PR: Pulmonary Regurgitation

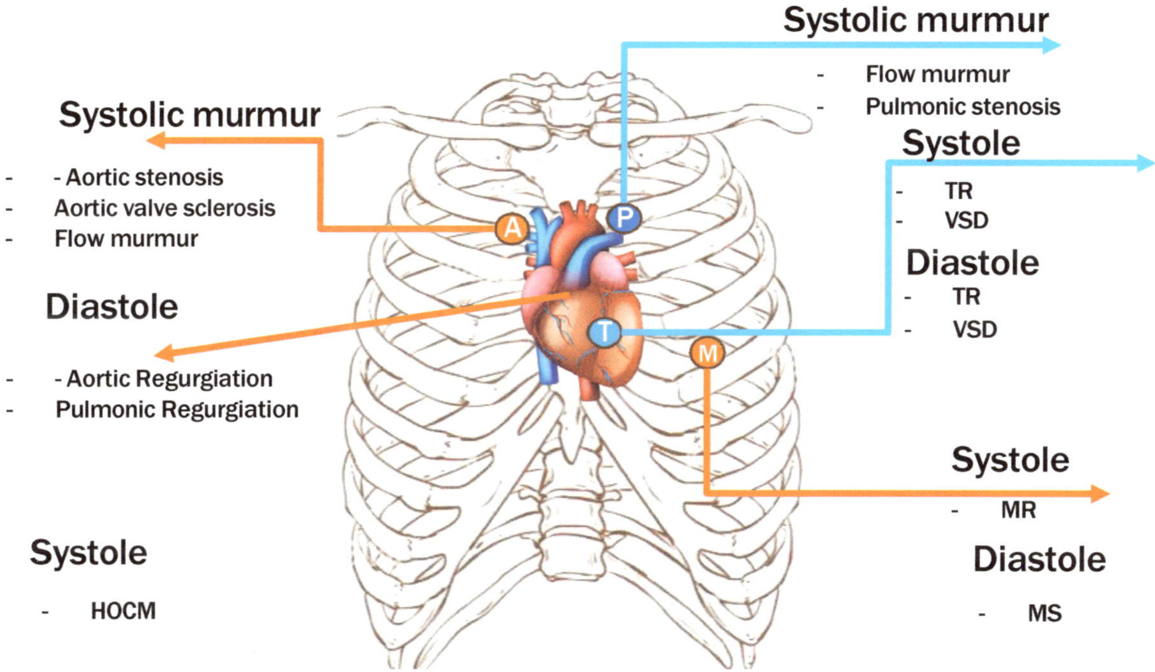

Chest Exam: Auscultation site

Bronchial – loud high pitched sounds around the trachea

Bronchovesicular – medium pictched sounds 2nd and 3rd IC space

Vesciular – soft and slow pitched – entirety of the lungs

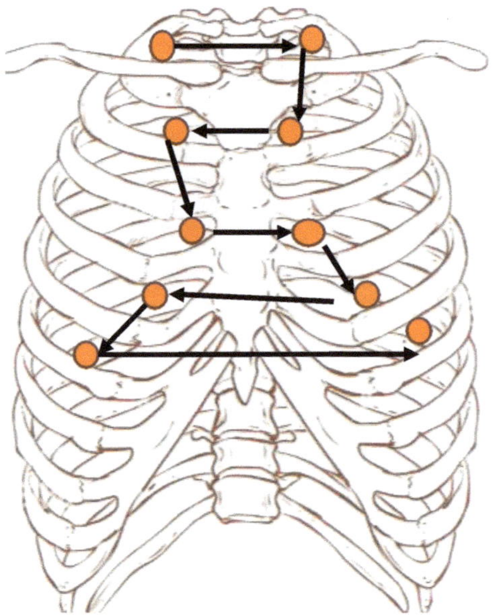

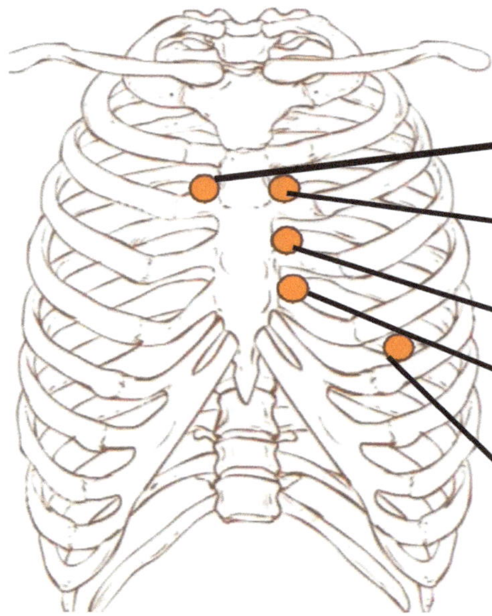

Aortic area – right of sternum 2nd IC space

Pulmonic area – Left of sternum – 2nd IC space

Erb's point left of sterum 3rd IC space

Tricuspid –Left of sterum 4th IC space

Mitral – Left sternum 5th IC space

Auscultation is essential for evaluating heart sounds and murmurs. Listen for S1 (closure of mitral/tricuspid valves) and S2 (closure of aortic/pulmonic valves) to assess rhythm and rate.
Identify any extra heart sounds like S3 or S4 gallops, which can indicate ventricular dysfunction or stiffness, respectively.

Systematically listen for murmurs across all five auscultatory areas (aortic, pulmonic, Erb's point, tricuspid, mitral), noting their timing (systolic/diastolic), intensity, pitch, quality, and radiation.

Use dynamic maneuvers (e.g., squatting, Valsalva, handgrip) to differentiate murmurs and assess their physiological significance.

Listen for pericardial rubs, which are scratchy, high-pitched sounds indicative of pericardial inflammation, often best heard with the patient leaning forward and holding their breath in expiration.

- **Right-sided murmurs get louder with Inspiration** (e.g., Tricuspid regurgitation, Pulmonic stenosis)
- **Left-sided murmurs get louder with Expiration** (e.g., Mitral regurgitation, Aortic stenosis, Aortic regurgitation, Mitral stenosis)

Radiation Patterns

These are classic findings used in OSCEs and clinical exams.

Aortic Stenosis (AS)
Radiation: To the carotids
Why: High-velocity jet through a narrowed aortic valve transmits up the aorta.

Mitral Regurgitation (MR)
Radiation: To the axilla
Why: Regurgitant jet directed laterally toward the left atrium.

Tricuspid Regurgitation (TR)
Radiation: To the right lower sternal border Often increases with inspiration (Carvallo's sign).

Aortic Regurgitation (AR)
Radiation: May radiate along the left sternal border; best heard at Erb's point.
Pulmonic Stenosis (PS)
Radiation: Toward the left shoulder/neck.

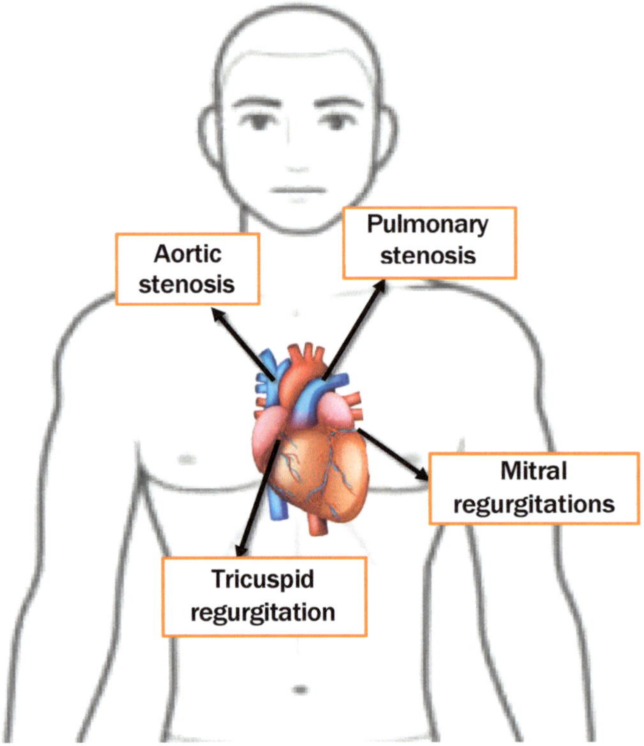

Quick Memory Aids:

AS → Carotids ("Aortic → Arteries of the neck")

MR → Left Axilla ("Mitral → Mammary area") PS

→ Left Shoulder ("Pulmonary → Periphery") TR →

Epigastrium ("Tricuspid → Tummy")

•Right-sided murmurs get louder with Inspiration (e.g., Tricuspid regurgitation, Pulmonic stenosis)
•Left-sided murmurs get louder with Expiration (e.g., Mitral regurgitation, Aortic stenosis, Aortic regurgitation, Mitral stenosis)

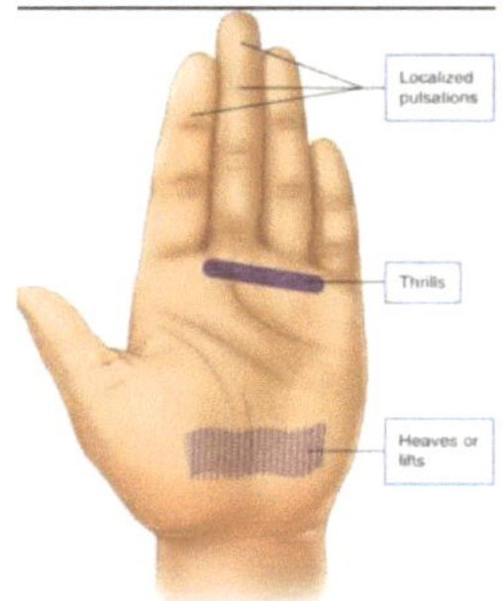

Inspection: Chest

Assess for skin changes such as pallor, cyanosis,Scars or rashes that might indicate systemic disease.

Look for signs of respiratory distress that could impact cardiac function, like increased work of breathing or use of accessory muscles.

Identify any visible venous distension (e.g., jugular venous distension) which can indicate right heart failure.

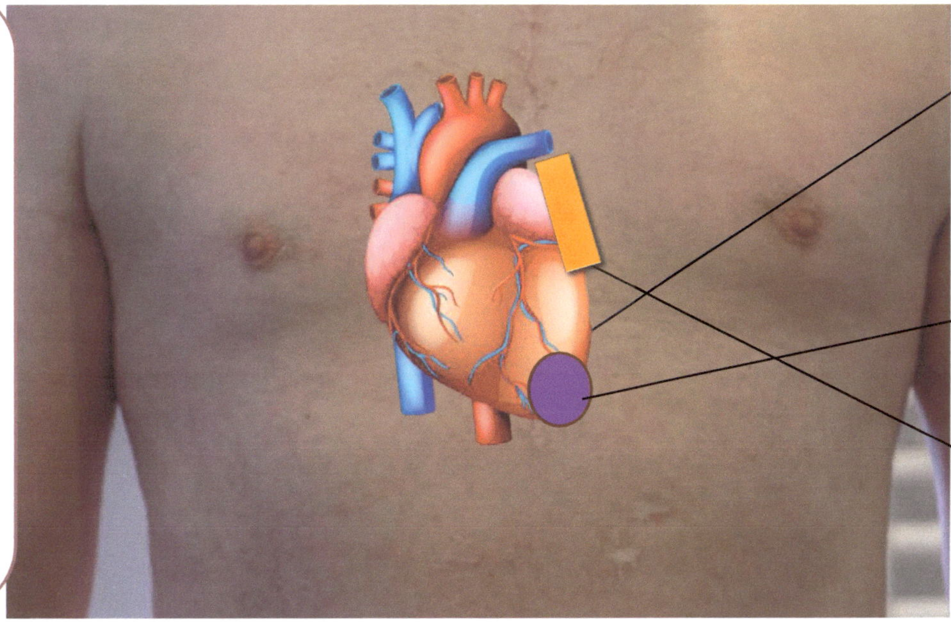

Precordial Pulsations: While a normal apical impulse (Point of Maximum Impulse, PMI) may sometimes be visible, prominent or widespread pulsations can indicate ventricular hypertrophy or dilation

Heaves or Thrills: These are sustained, forceful outward thrusts of the chest wall, often visible or palpable, and suggest significant ventricular hypertrophy

A left parasternal heave is often associated with right ventricular hypertrophy, while an apical heave suggests left ventricular hypertrophy

Look for conditions such as pectus excavatum (hollowed chest), barrel chest (associated with emphysema and hyperinflation), kyphosis (forward bending of the spine), and scoliosis (lateral spinal curvature)

Inspection: legs

nspect for edema (swelling), particularly pitting edema, which can be a sign of right-sided heart failure. Observe for skin discoloration (e.g., hyperpigmentation, hemosiderin staining) or trophic changes indicative of chronic venous insufficiency or

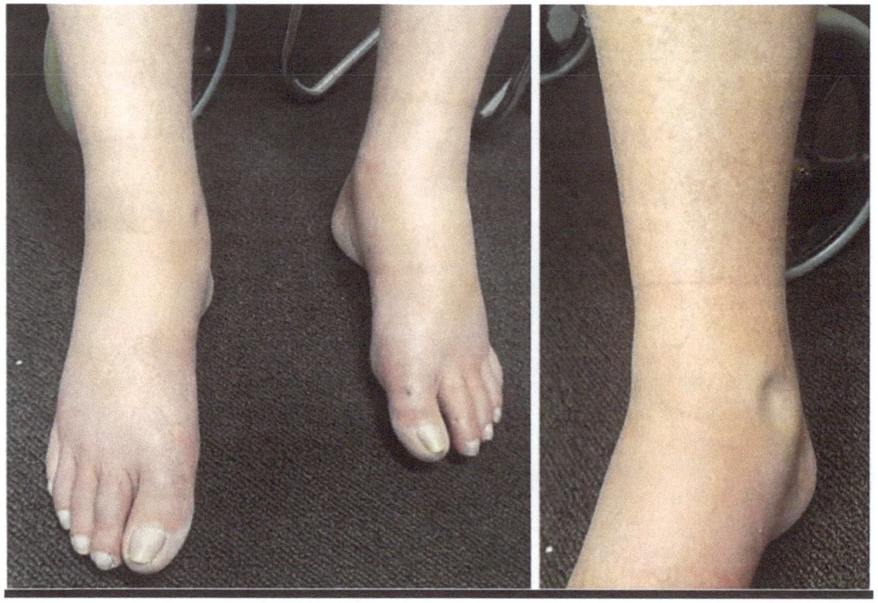

peripheral arterial disease. Look for varicose veins or other signs of venous stasis. Check for hair loss, shiny skin, or ulcers on the lower extremities, suggesting peripheral arterial disease. Assess for any asymmetry in leg size or color, which could point to deep vein thrombosis or other vascular

Observe for pallor (unusual paleness) of the skin and mucous membranes, suggesting anemia or poor perfusion.

Check for central cyanosis (bluish discoloration of lips and tongue), indicating severe hypoxemia.

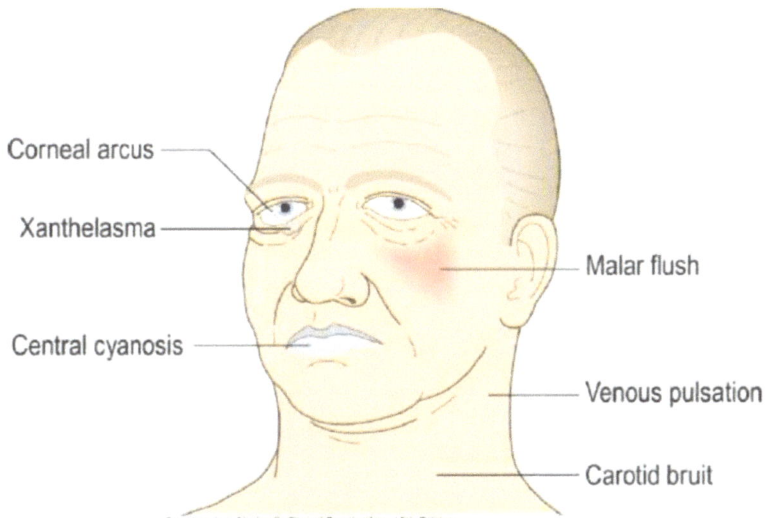

Look for xanthelasma (yellowish plaques around the eyelids) or corneal arcus (a white, gray, or blue opaque ring in the corneal margin), which can be signs of hyperlipidemia.

Assess for malar flush (reddish-purple discoloration of the cheeks), often associated with mitral stenosis.

Note any facial asymmetry or signs of stroke, which can be a complication of cardiac conditions like atrial fibrillation.

Inspection: hands

Check for clubbing (bulbous enlargement of fingertips), which can be associated with congenital heart disease or endocarditis.

Observe for cyanosis (bluish discoloration) of the nail beds or fingertips, indicating poor oxygenation.

Look for splinter hemorrhages (small, linear red-brown streaks under the nails), a sign of infective endocarditis.

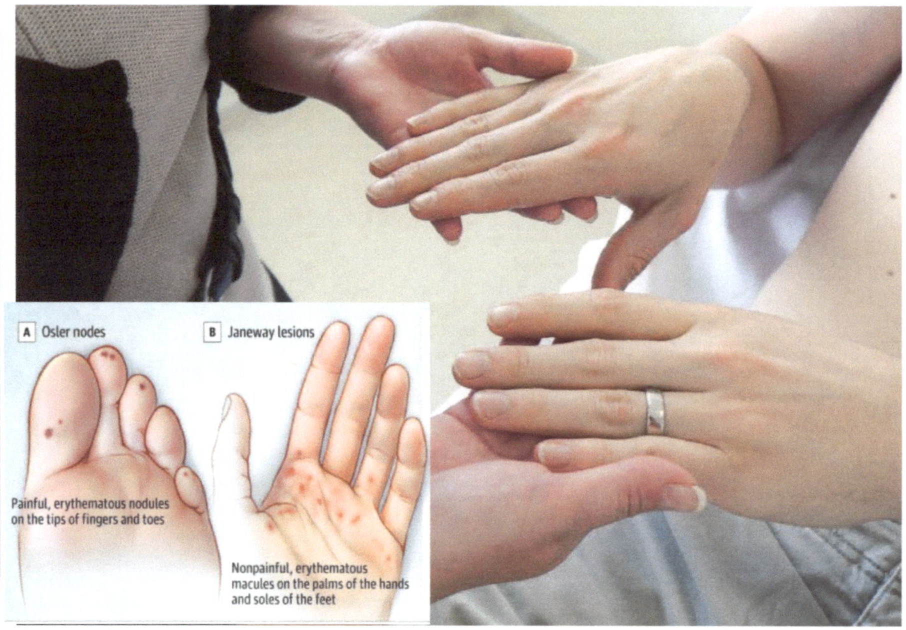

Assess for Janeway lesions (painless, erythematous macules on palms/soles) or Osler's nodes (tender, subcutaneous nodules on fingertips/toes), both associated with endocarditis.

Note any signs of peripheral vascular disease, such as trophic changes, pallor, or absent hair growth

Summarising

Synthesize Key Findings: After completing the physical exam (inspection, palpation, auscultation), mentally or verbally summarize the most pertinent positive and negative findings. This isn't a re-listing of everything, but a concise overview of what's clinically significant.

Focus on Relevant Systems: While the exam might touch on general appearance, the summary should primarily focus on cardiovascular findings, linking them to the patient's presenting complaint.

Formulate a Working Diagnosis (if appropriate): Based on your findings, consider if a preliminary diagnosis or a differer diagnosis can be formulated. This demonstrates clinical reasoning.

Identify Next Steps: Briefly outline what further investigations (e.g., ECG, echocardiogram, blood tests) or management strategies might be necessary based on your summary.

Communicate Clearly and Concisely: Present your summary in a structured and easy-to-understand manner. Avoid jargon where possible, especially when speaking to a patient.

Patient-Centered Approach: When ending the exam with the patient, ensure your summary addresses their

Resp Exam

- **Introduction**
  - Wash hands and don PPE if appropriate.
  - Introduce yourself (name and role).
  - Confirm patient identity (name and DOB).
  - Explain the procedure in simple terms.
  - Obtain consent.
- **General Inspection**
  - *Signs of respiratory distress*: nasal flaring, accessory muscle use, tripod position.
  - *Cyanosis*: bluish discoloration of lips or extremities.
  - *Cough*: dry or productive.
  - *Wheeze*: audible sounds.
  - *Scars, sputum pots, oxygen equipment.*
- **Face and neck:**
  - Inspect eyes for *conjunctival pallor*.
  - Inspect mouth for *central cyanosis*.
  - Assess *tracheal position*:
  - Deviation suggests pneumothorax or lung collapse
- **Chest inpection**
  - Look for:
  - *Scars, deformities, asymmetry.*
  - *Chest wall movement* and *intercostal recession*.
- **Palpation**
  - Palpation
  - Assess *chest expansion* (anterior and posterior).
  - Palpate for *tactile vocal fremitus* (optional).
- **Percussion**
  - Percuss:
  - *Anterior, lateral, and posterior chest.*
  - Compare sides.
  - Note dullness (e.g., consolidation, effusion) or hyperresonance (e.g., pneumothorax).

Resp Exam

Auscultation:
- Ask patient to breathe deeply through mouth.
- Auscultate:
- *Supraclavicular, anterior, lateral, and posterior areas.*
- Listen for: *Normal breath sounds.*
- *Added sounds:* crackles, wheeze, stridor.
- *Vocal resonance:* increased in consolidation, decreased in effusion. Ask patient to breathe deeply through mouth.,

Posterior chest
- Repeat inspection, palpation, percussion, and auscultation on the back.

Lower Limbs
- InInspect for *peripheral edema* (suggestive of cor pulmonale).
- Check *calves for swelling or tenderness* (DVT signs).

To complete the exam
- Suggest:
- *Reviewing observation chart* (especially oxygen saturation).
- *Measuring peak flow* (if asthma suspected).
- *Chest X-ray or sputum culture* if indicated.

Palpation
- Palpation
- Assess *chest expansion* (anterior and posterior).
- Palpate for *tactile vocal fremitus* (optional).

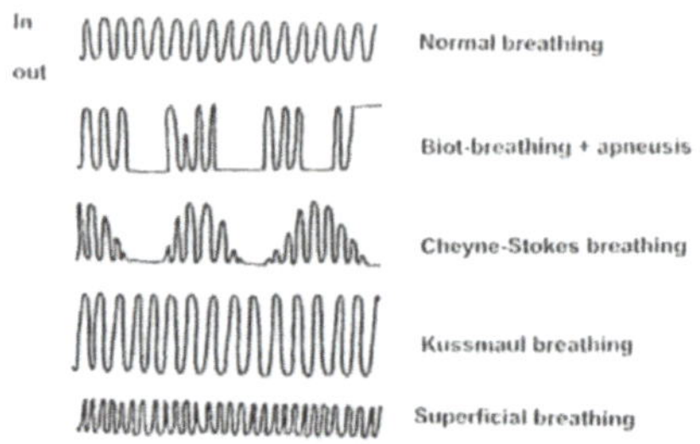

Observe the patient's general appearance and comfort level, noting any signs of respiratory distress such as labored breathing, use of accessory muscles (e.g., sternocleidomastoids, scalenes), or a "tripod position."

.

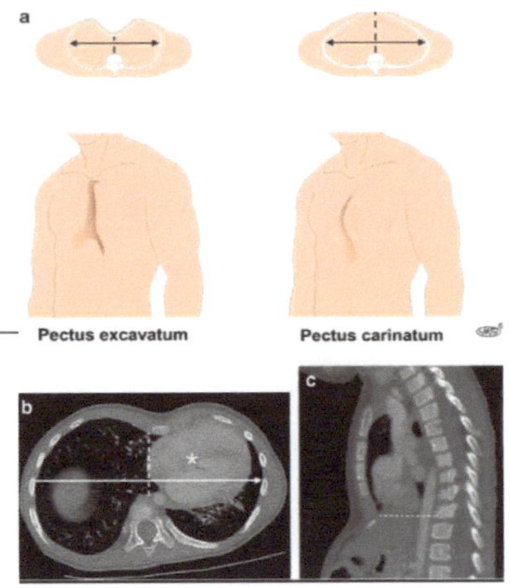

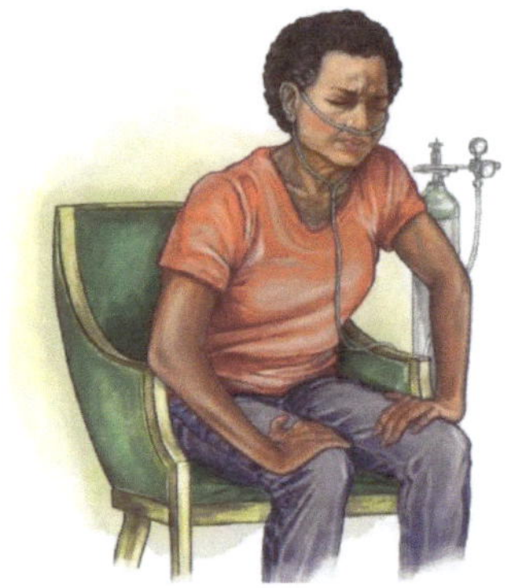

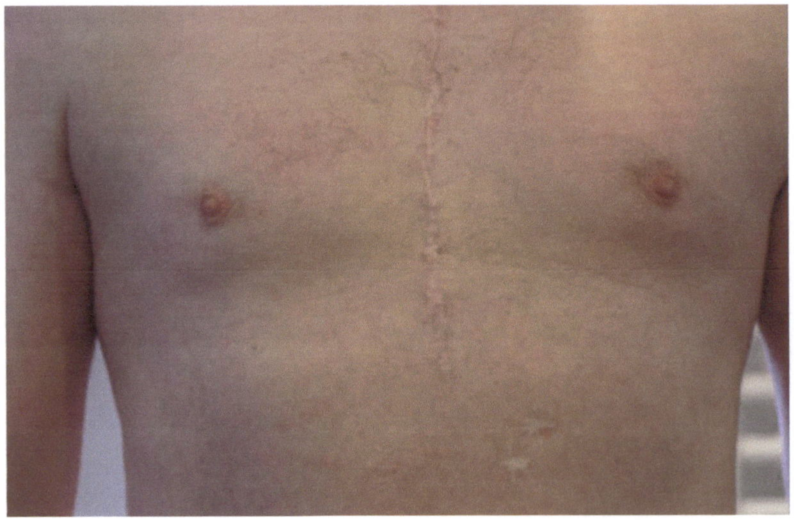

Assess the patient's breathing pattern, Inspect the chest wall for deformities, such as pectus excavatum (funnel chest), pectus carinatum (pigeon chest), kyphosis, scoliosis, or a "barrel chest" (increased anterior-posterior diameter, often seen in COPD).

Assess the patient's breathing pattern, including rate, rhythm, depth, and symmetry. Look for abnormal patterns like Kussmaul breathing (deep, rapid), Cheyne-Stokes (waxing and waning), or paradoxical breathing.

Look for signs of cyanosis (bluish discoloration of lips, nail beds) which indicates hypoxemia, and clubbing of the fingers, which can be associated with chronic respiratory or cardiac conditions.

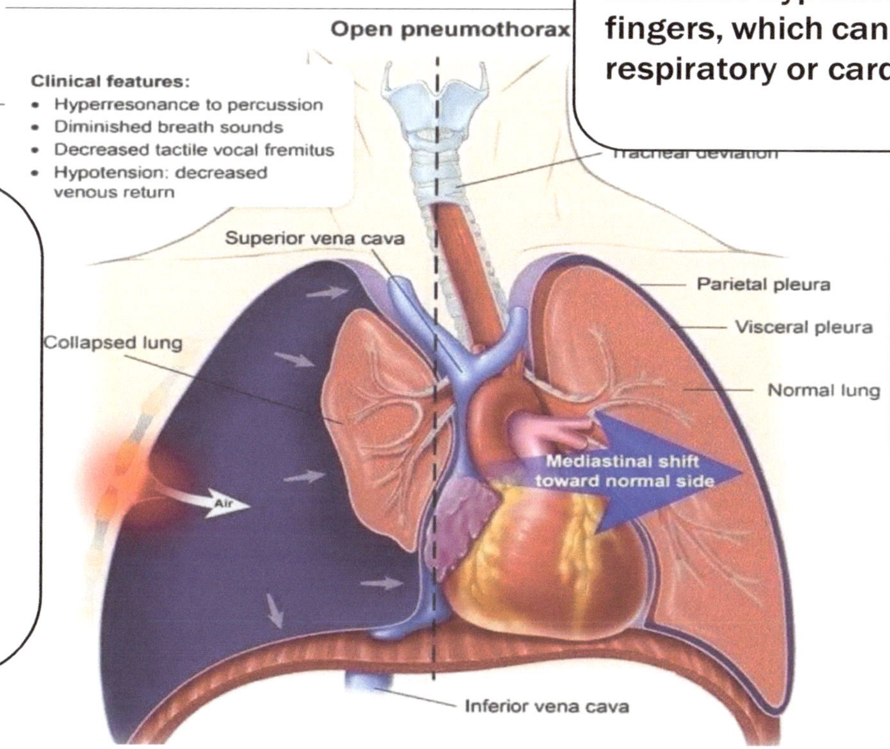

Assess for Hoover's sign (paradoxical inward movement of the lower intercostal spaces during inspiration) and Dahl's sign (hyperpigmentation/bruising above the knees from constant "tenting" position), both associated with severe COPD

Observe for tracheal deviation, which can indicate conditions like pneumothorax or atelectasis.

Perform systematic percussion over the anterior, lateral, and posterior chest walls, comparing symmetrical areas to identify differences in sound. (percussion notes)

Identify areas of resonance, which is the normal sound heard over healthy, air-filled lung tissue. – (low hollow and longer lasting)

Note areas of dullness, which suggests underlying consolidation (e.g., pneumonia), pleural effusion (fluid), or tumor. (soft and short)

Identify areas of hyperresonance, which indicates excessive air, as seen in pneumothorax or emphysema (Higher booming lasts longer)

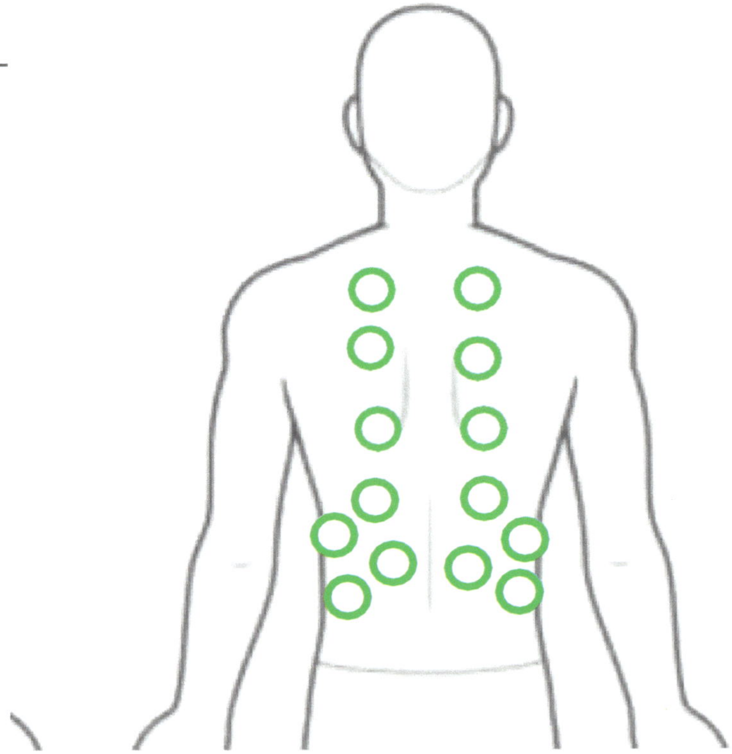

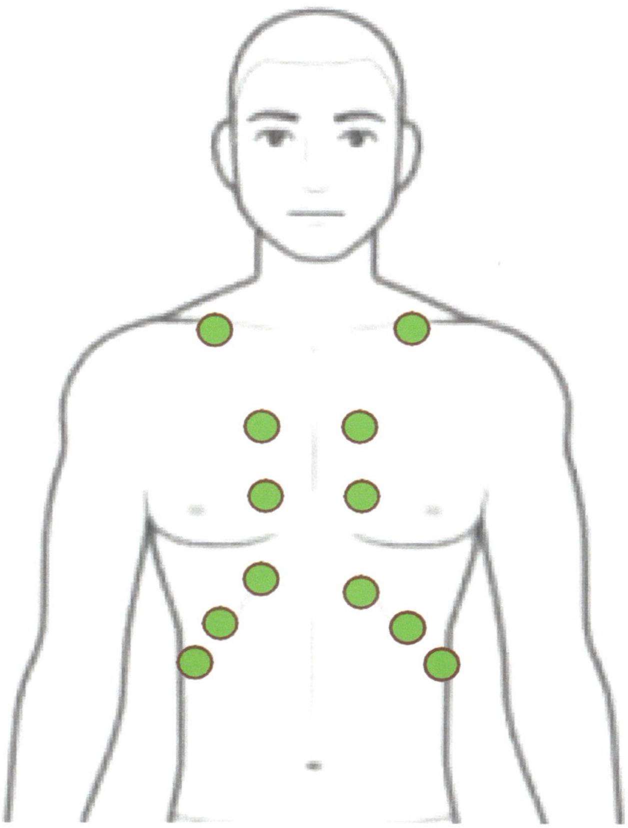

Determine diaphragmatic excursion by percussing downwards from resonance to dullness during both inspiration and expiration, noting the distance the diaphragm moves. Reduced excursion can indicate pleural effusion or hyperinflation.

Assess for cardiac dullness, a fist-sized area to the left of the sternum, which may be absent in severe emphysema due to lung hyperinflation.

Check Traube's space (over the gastric bubble) for hyperresonance; loss of this can indicate splenomegaly or left pleural effusion.

Auscultation – Breath sounds

Breath Sounds (Normal): Listen for vesicular breath sounds (soft, low-pitched, heard over most lung fields, inspiration longer than expiration) and bronchial breath sounds (loud, high-pitched, heard over trachea, expiration longer than inspiration)

Adventitious Sounds (Added Sounds): Identify and characterize abnormal sounds

- Crackles (Rales): Discontinuous, popping sounds, often heard during inspiration. Fine crackles (like hair rubbing) suggest interstitial disease or early pulmonary edema. Coarse crackles (like Velcro) suggest secretions in larger airways or pulmonary edema
- Wheezes: Continuous, high-pitched, musical sounds, usually expiratory, caused by narrowed airways (bronchospasm, edema, foreign body)
- Rhonchi: Continuous, low-pitched, snoring or gurgling sounds, often heard on expiration, caused by secretions in larger airways
- Stridor: A harsh, high-pitched, inspiratory sound, indicating upper airway obstruction (e.g., croup, epiglottitis, foreign body)
- Pleural Friction Rub: A creaking or grating sound, like walking on fresh snow, caused by inflamed pleural surfaces rubbing together

Sounds: Assess for abnormal transmission of spoken words

- Bronchophony: Increased clarity and loudness of spoken words (e.g., "ninety-nine") over consolidated areas.
- Egophony: A nasal or bleating quality to spoken "eee" sounds, which changes to "aaa" over consolidated lung.
- Whispered Pectoriloquy: Increased clarity of whispered words over consolidated areas.

- Crackles (Rales): Discontinuous, popping sounds, often heard during inspiration. Fine crackles (like hair rubbing) suggest interstitial disease or early pulmonary edema. Coarse crackles (like Velcro) suggest secretions in larger airways or pulmonary edema
- Wheezes: Continuous, high-pitched, musical sounds, usually expiratory, caused by narrowed airways (bronchospasm, edema, foreign body)

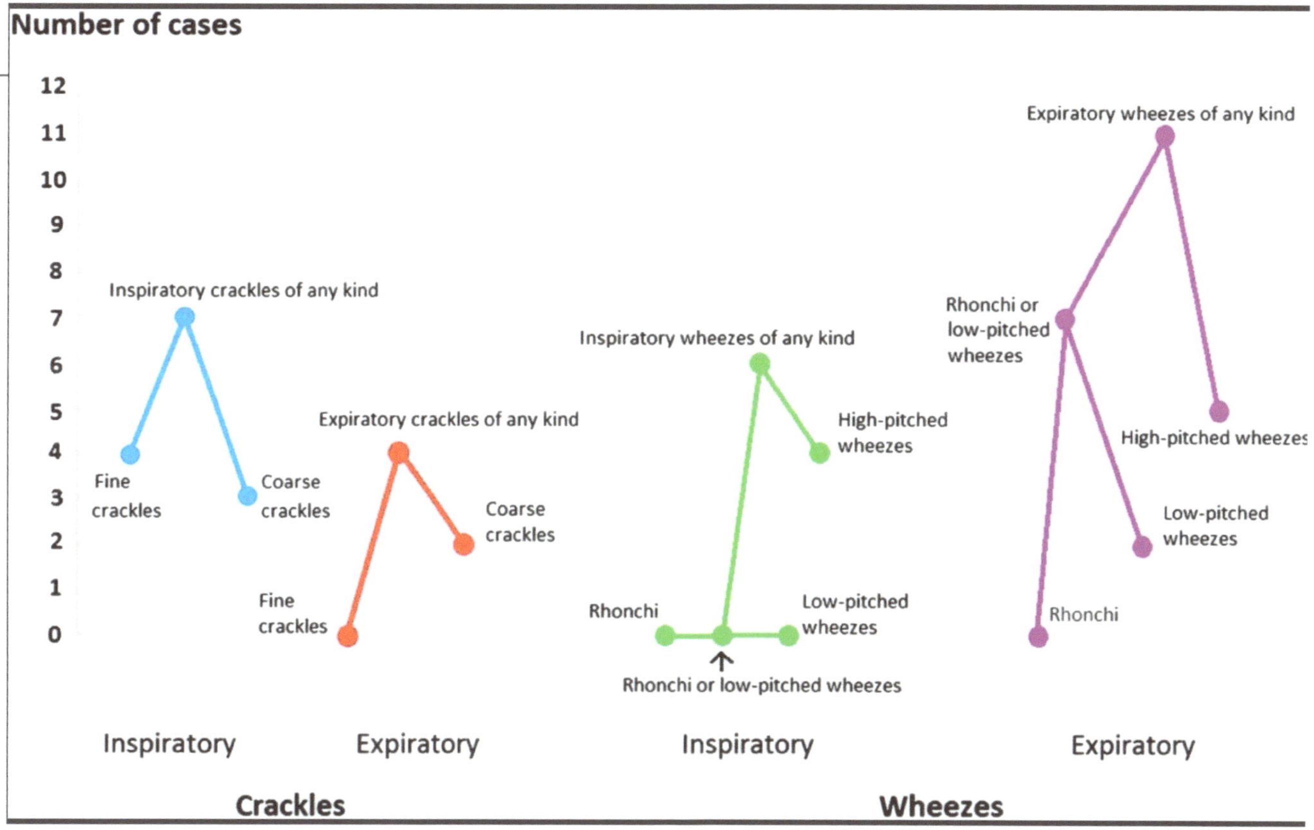

Crackles: Discontinuous, popping sounds, often heard during inspiration. Fine crackles (like hair rubbing) suggest interstitial disease or early pulmonary edema. Coarse crackles (like Velcro) suggest secretions in larger airways

RHONCI: Continuous, low-pitched, snoring or gurgling sounds, often heard on expiration, caused by secretions in larger airways

WHEEZING: Continuous, high-pitched, musical sounds, usually expiratory, caused by narrowed airways (bronchospasm, edema, foreign body)

STRIDOR: A harsh, high-pitched, inspiratory sound, indicating upper airway obstruction (e.g., croup, epiglottitis, foreign body)

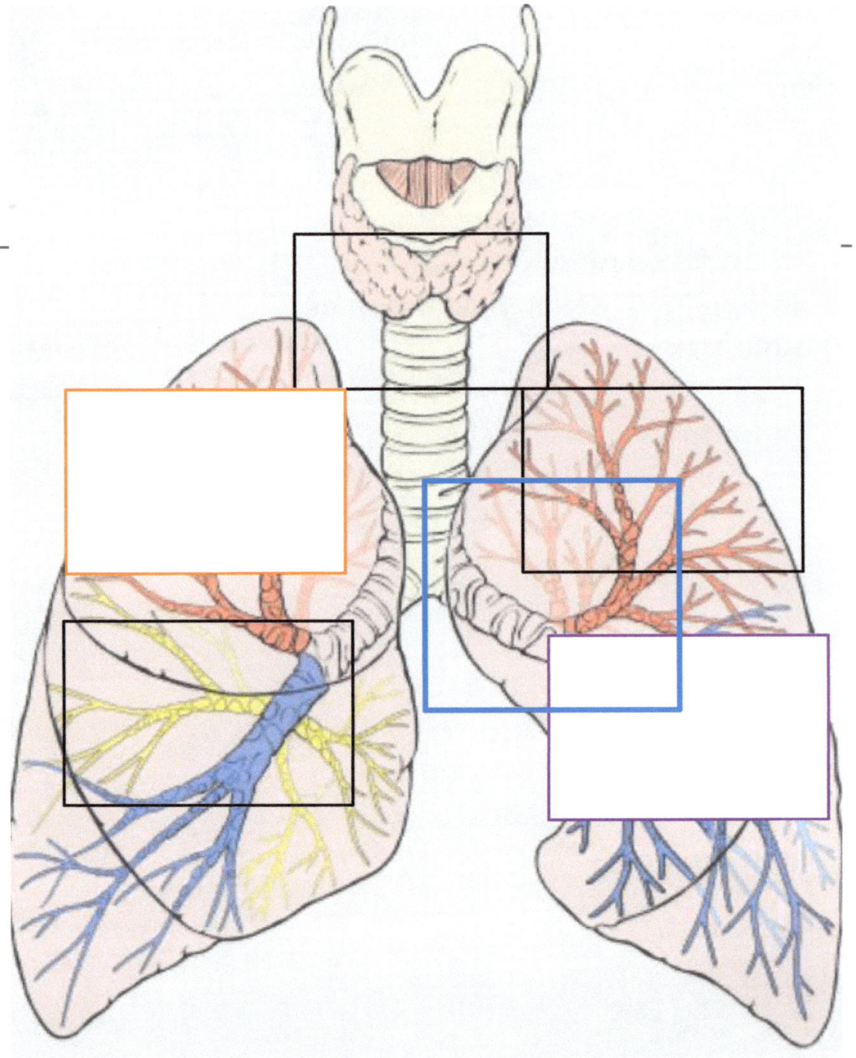

Assessing vocal fremitus

Sounds: Assess for abnormal transmission of spoken words

- Bronchophony: Increased clarity and loudness of spoken words (e.g., "ninety-nine") over consolidated areas.
- Egophony: A nasal or bleating quality to spoken "eee" sounds, which changes to "aaa" over consolidated lung.
- Whispered Pectoriloquy: Increased clarity of whispered words over consolidated areas.

Heart Sounds: Listen for a loud S2 over the pulmonary valve area, which can signify pulmonary hypertension

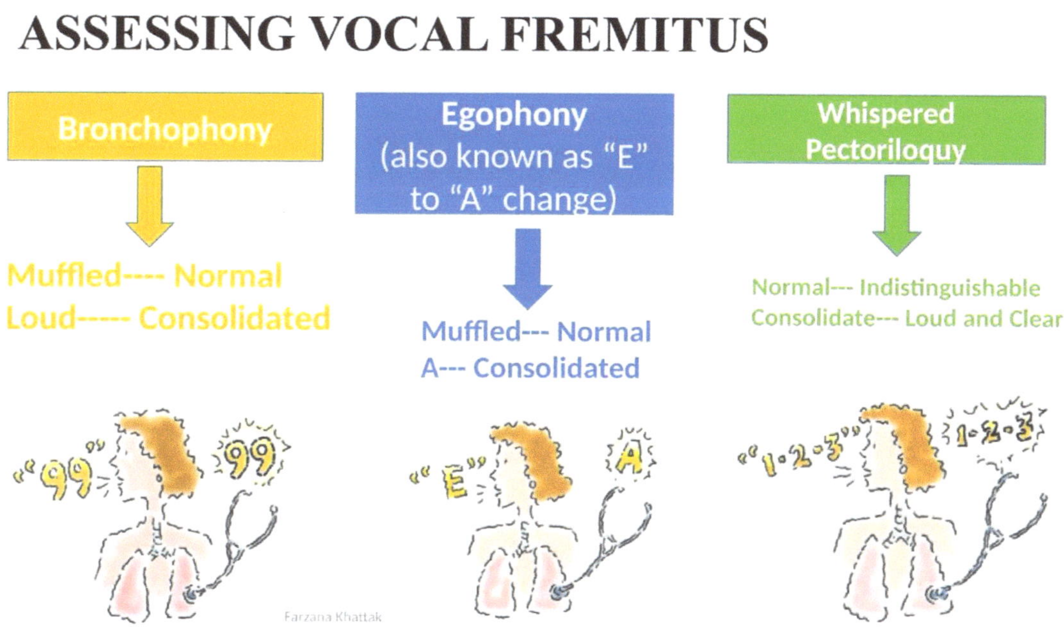

Legs: Examine the legs for peripheral oedema by pressing over the tibia (suggests cor pulmonale) and feel the calves for swelling or tenderness, which could indicate deep vein thrombosis (DVT).

Further Investigations: After the physical examination, consider reviewing the observations chart (especially oxygen saturations) and measuring peak flow (if the patient is asthmatic). Summarize findings and suggest further investigations based on the clinical picture.

The patient, a 68-year-old male, presented with shortness of breath and a chronic cough. On examination, he exhibited pursed-lip breathing and a barrel chest, consistent with chronic obstructive pulmonary disease (COPD). Clubbing was noted on his fingers, and bilateral fine inspiratory crackles were auscultated at the lung bases, alongside diminished breath sounds throughout both lung fields. Percussion revealed hyperresonance over both lungs, and tactile fremitus was reduced bilaterally. His JVP was mildly elevated, and a right ventricular heave was palpable, suggesting potential cor pulmonale.

Neuro Exam – Upper limb

Tone	Ask patient to relax arm.	Roll forearm, flex/extend elbow and wrist.	Look for spasticity or rigidity.			
Power	Shoulder abduction/adduction.	Elbow flexion/extension.	Wrist extension/flexion.	Finger extension/flexion.	Finger abduction (ulnar nerve).	Thumb opposition (median nerve).
Reflexes	Biceps (C5/6)	Triceps (C7)	Brachioradialis (C6)	Hoffmann's reflex (if indicated)		
Coordination	Finger-to-nose test.	Rapid alternating movements.				
Sensation:	Light touch, pinprick, vibration, proprioception.	Compare sides and dermatomes.				

General Inspection
Observe for:

Posture, gait, involuntary movements (e.g., tremors, chorea).
Muscle wasting or fasciculations.
Assistive devices: walking aids, splints.
Speech abnormalities.

Neuro Exam – Lower Limb exam

- **Tone**
  - Roll leg, lift knee, assess ankle tone.
  - Check for *clonus* at ankle.
- **Power**
  - Hip flexion/extension.
  - Knee flexion/extension.
  - Ankle dorsiflexion/plant arflexion
  - Toe extension
- **Reflexes**
  - Knee jerk (L3/4)
  - Ankle jerk (S1/2)
  - Plantar reflex (Babinski's sign)
- **Coordination**
  - Heel to shin
- **Sensation**
  - Light touch, pinprick, vibration, proprioception.
  - Test dermatomes and compare sides.
- **Gait and cerebellar functions:**
  - Observe normal walking.
  - Heel-to-toe walking.
  - Romberg test.
  - Tandem gait.
  - Turn quickly – assess balance

To Complete the Examination Suggest:

- Full cognitive assessment (e.g., MMSE).
- Neuroimaging if indicated.
- Blood tests or lumbar puncture if relevant.

The initial steps of a neurological examination are essential for setting the stage and gathering preliminary observations. This begins with standard introductory procedures, often remembered by the acronym WIIPPPE: Wash your hands, Introduce yourself, Identify the patient, obtain Permission, ask about Pain, Position the patient, and Ensure adequate Exposure.

Following this, a thorough inspection is performed, which is particularly vital in neurology. This involves observing the patient's overall presentation, including their handshake (which can reveal issues like weakness or myotonia), any assistive devices around the bed (e.g., wheelchair, catheter bag, spirometer), and the patient's posture, symmetry, muscle atrophy, and fasciculations

Closer Inspection: Observe each muscle group for size, shape, and symmetry, noting any atrophy (indicating disuse) or hypertrophy (potentially compensatory).

Look for fasciculations, especially in the deltoid.
Tone: Assess muscle tone by passively moving the patient's joints, particularly the wrist, through their range of motion. Note if tone is decreased (hypotonia, often in lower motor neuron lesions) or increased (hypertonia, often in upper motor neuron lesions). Differentiate between spasticity (velocity-dependent, "clasp-knife" phenomenon) and rigidity (constant resistance, "lead-pipe" or "cog-wheel" if tremor is present).

Feature	Spasticity	Rigidity
Definition	Velocity-dependent increase in muscle tone due to hyperactive stretch reflex.	Velocity-independent increase in muscle tone affecting both flexors and extensors.
Cause	Upper Motor Neuron (UMN) lesions (e.g., stroke, cerebral palsy, multiple sclerosis, spinal cord injury).	Basal ganglia disorders (e.g., Parkinson's disease).

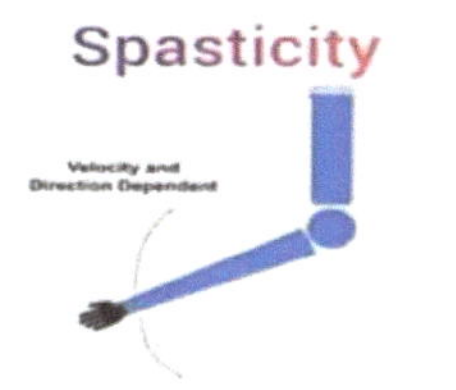

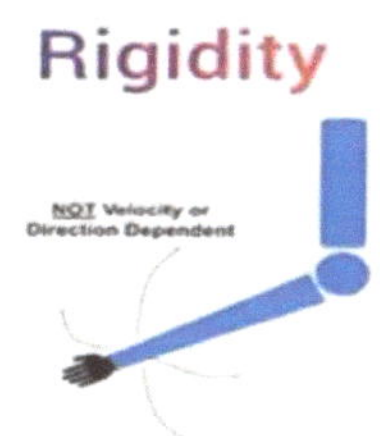

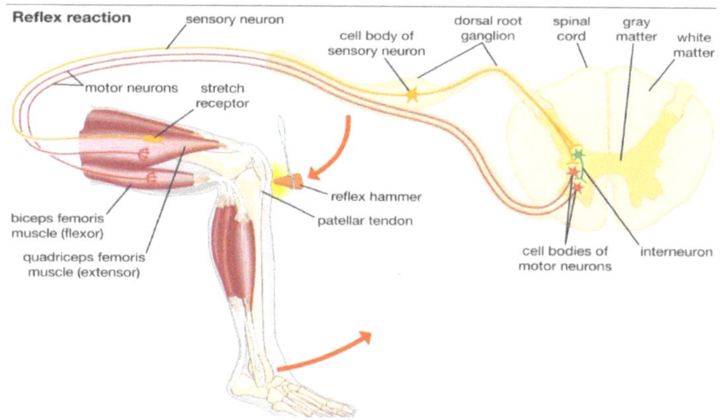

Power: Evaluate muscle strength using the Medical Research Council (MRC) grading scale from 0 (absent contraction) to 5 (full strength) Test specific muscle groups and, if time is limited, assess grip strength and proximal/distal movements

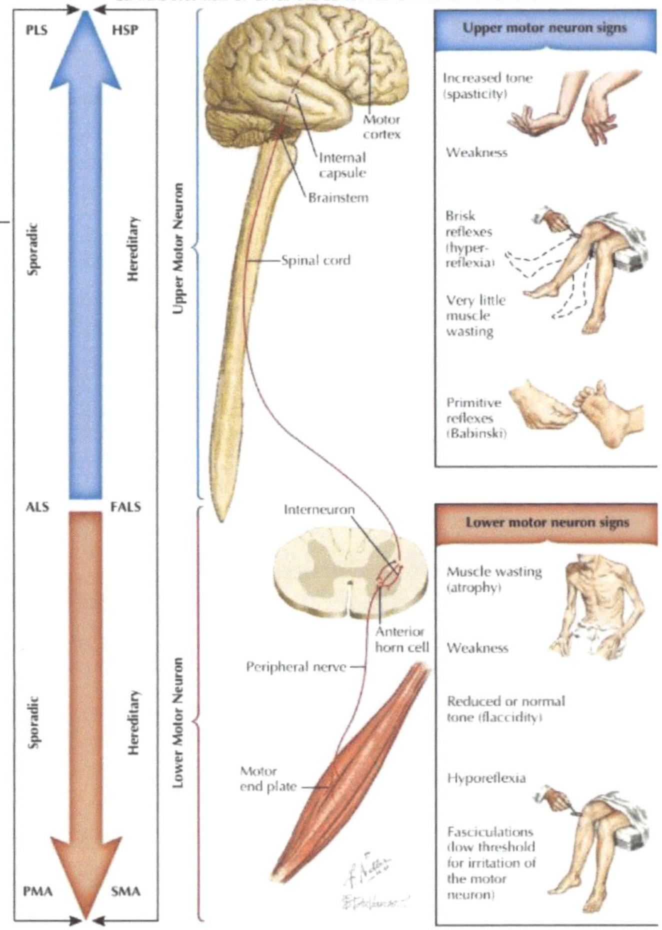

Grade	Muscle Power
5	Normal power
4	Active movement against resistance and gravity
3	Active movement against gravity but not resistance
2	Active movement possible only with gravity eliminated
1	Flicker or trace of contraction
0	No contraction

Reflexes: Test deep tendon reflexes (biceps C5/6, triceps C7/8, brachioradialis C6) to differentiate between upper and lower motor neuron lesions. Reinforce reflexes using Jendrassik's manoeuvre if they are absence. Describe reflexes as hyporeflexic, normal, or brisk (e.g., +, ++, +++).

Coordination: Assess fine motor skills modulated by the basal ganglia and cerebellum. This includes the finger-nose test (looking for past pointing and intention tremor) and dysdiadochokinesis (rapid alternating movements, like clapping hands

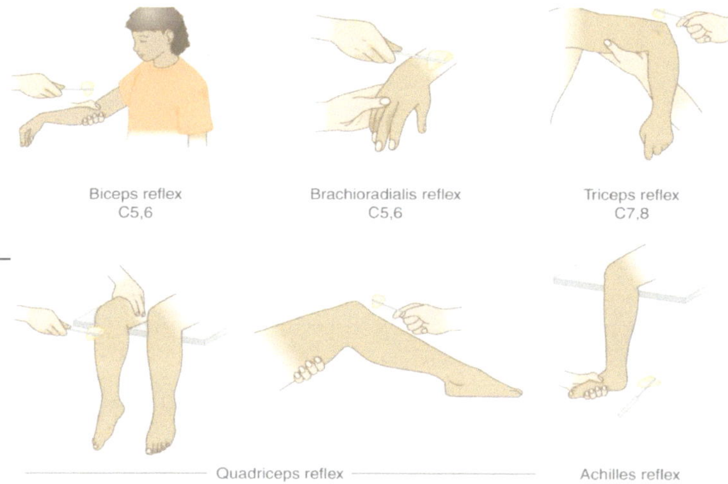

Coordination: The heel-shin test is used to assess lower limb coordination, looking for the heel sliding off the shin

Gait: Observe the patient's gait for posture, arm swing, step size, base width, and ability to walk on toes or heels. Identify pathological gaits such as ataxic (broad-based), shuffling (festinating), tilted, or high-stepping.

Romberg's Test: This test assesses proprioception. The patient stands with feet together and arms outstretched, then closes their eyes.

A positive Romberg's sign (falling with eyes closed but not open) indicates sensory ataxia, while unsteadiness with both eyes open and closed suggests cerebellar dysfunction

Romberg Test

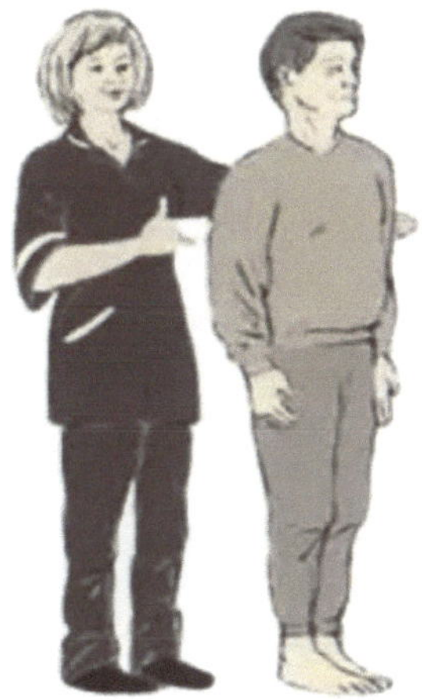

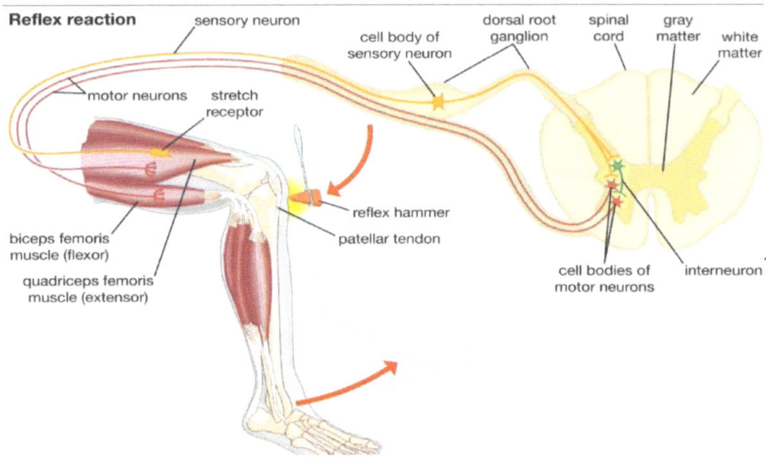

This diagram illustrates the fundamental components of the knee-jerk reflex, also known as the patellar reflex. When the patellar tendon is tapped with a reflex hammer, stretch receptors in the quadriceps muscle are activated. These receptors send signals via sensory neurons to the spinal cord, specifically entering through the dorsal root ganglion. Within the spinal cord's gray matter, the signal is processed and immediately relayed through motor neurons back to the quadriceps muscle, causing it to contract and produce the characteristic leg kick. The diagram also shows the inhibition of the opposing muscle (biceps femoris), ensuring smooth extension. This process is a classic example of a monosynaptic reflex, where the sensory and motor neurons communicate directly without involving the brain.

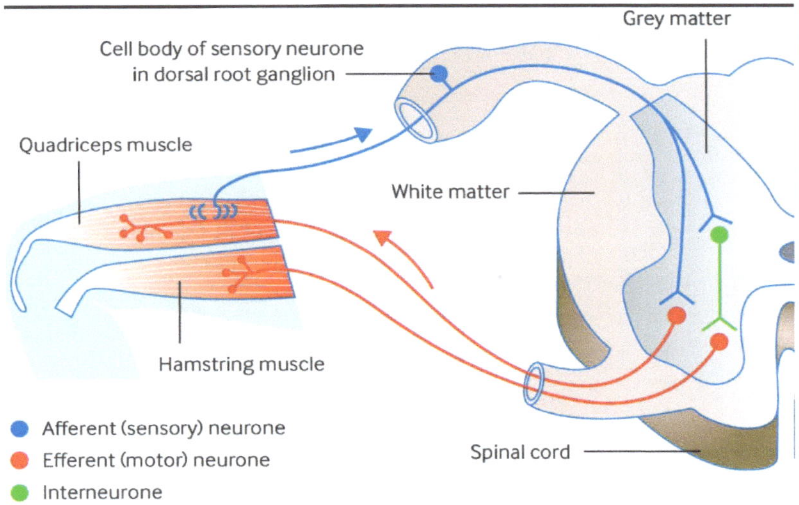

This diagram provides a more anatomically detailed view of the neural circuitry involved in the patellar reflex. It color-codes the different types of neurons: blue for afferent (sensory), red for efferent (motor), and green for interneurons. The sensory neuron originates in the quadriceps muscle and carries the signal to the spinal cord, where its cell body resides in the dorsal root ganglion. Inside the spinal cord, the signal is transmitted to a motor neuron that activates the quadriceps, while an interneuron simultaneously inhibits the hamstring (biceps femoris) to allow unopposed extension. The diagram highlights the roles of gray and white matter in signal transmission and emphasizes the reciprocal inhibition mechanism that ensures coordinated muscle movement during reflex actions.

General Assessment: Ask about numbness or tingling. Begin by lightly touching the upper chest and then systematically test limbs, asking the patient to identify the side touched and if sensation feels equal.

Dermatomes: Test specific dermatomal areas to localize lesions. Key upper limb dermatomes include C6 (thumb), C7 (middle finger), C8 (little finger). Lower limb dermatomes include L4 (medial malleolus), L5 (big toe), and S1 (heel)

Other Sensory Modalities:

- Pain: Use a sharp and blunt object (e.g., neuro-tip) to test pain discrimination
- Temperature: Can be assessed with a cold object like a metal tuning fork
- Vibration: Test on bony prominences, asking the patient to indicate when they stop feeling the vibration
- Proprioception: Assess joint position sense, starting at the most distal joint (e.g., distal interphalangeal joint) and moving proximally if deficits are found

Mental state exam.

The mental status examination assesses cognitive functions and emotional state, providing insight into higher cortical function.

Appearance and Behavior: Observe grooming, posture, eye contact, and any unusual movements.

Speech: Note rate, rhythm, volume, and clarity of speech.

Mood and Affect: Inquire about mood and observe (emotional expression). affect

Thought Process and Content: Assess logical flow of thoughts, presence of delusions, hallucinations, or obsessions.

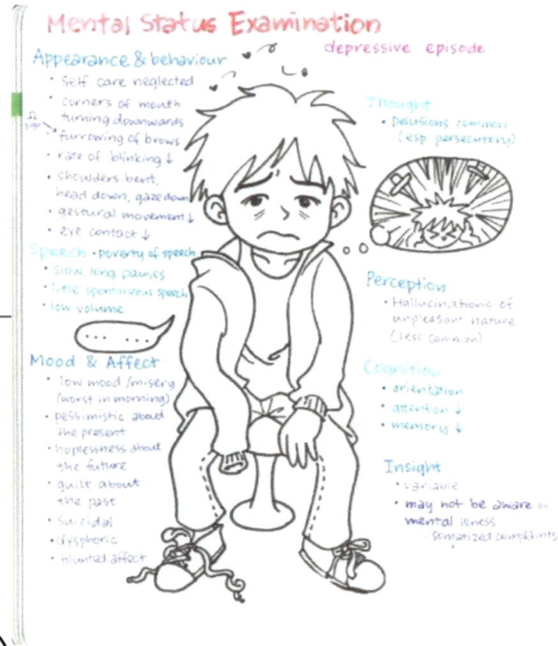

Cognitive Function:

Orientation: Test awareness of person, place, and time.

Attention and Concentration: Assess ability to focus (e.g., serial sevens, spelling "world" backward).

Memory: Test immediate, recent, and remote memory.

Language: Assess comprehension, naming, repetition, reading, and writing

Visuospatial Skills: Evaluate ability to copy figures or draw a clock

Executive Function: Assess planning, problem-solving, and abstract reasoning

Insight and Judgment: Evaluate the patient's understanding of their condition and ability to make sound decisions

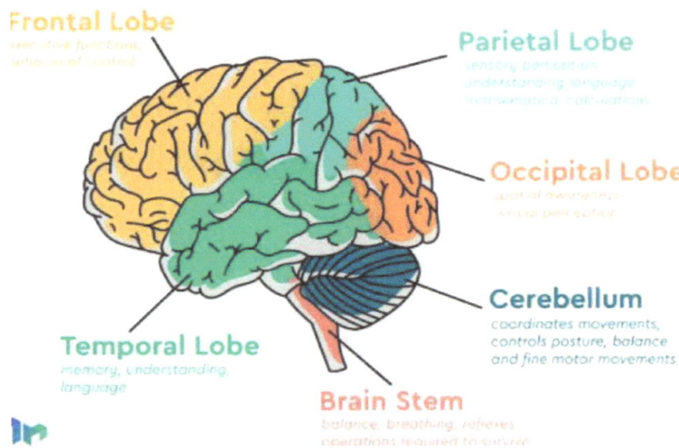

Knee exam

Geneeral Inspection
- *Gait* (if possible): limping, antalgic gait.
- *Posture and alignment*: valgus/varus deformity.
- *Swelling*: effusion, bursitis.
- *Scars*: previous surgery or trauma.
- *Muscle wasting*: especially quadriceps.
- *Skin changes*: redness, bruising, rashes.

Inspection
- Ask about pain before touching.
- Palpate for:
- *Temperature*: compare both knees.
- *Effusion*: sweep test or patellar tap.
- *Joint line tenderness*: medial and lateral.
- *Patella*: mobility and tenderness.
- *Quadriceps tendon and tibial tuberosity.*
- *Collateral ligaments*: medial (MCL) and lateral (LCL).
- *Popliteal fossa*: Baker's cyst or masses.

Rane of motion
- *Active and passive flexion/exten sion.*
- Normal range: ~0° extension to ~135° flexion.

Ligament stability test:
- Anterior Cruciate Ligament (ACL):
- *Anterior drawer test.*
- *Lachman's test* (more sensitive).
- Posterior Cruciate Ligament (PCL):
- *Posterior drawer test.*

Other ligaments
- Medial Collateral Ligament (MCL):
- *Valgus stress test.*
- Lateral Collateral Ligament (LCL):
- *Varus stress test.*

Meniscal test
- *McMurray's test*: flexion + rotation + extension.
- *Apley's grind test* (if patient prone).

Patellar test:
- *Patellar apprehension test*: lateral displacement.
- *Clarke's test*: patellofemoral pain.

Ask patient to:
Stand and walk (if safe).
Squat (if tolerated).
Observe for pain, instability, or crepitus.

To Complete the Examination
Suggest:
- *Examination of hip and ankle* (joint above and below).
- *Neurovascular assessment of the limb.*
- *Imaging*: X-ray, MRI if indicated.

t: Observe the patient's walking ern for any antalgic (pain-avoiding) gait, ing, or abnormal weight-bearing. A delenburg gait, for instance, might est hip pathology but can indirectly t knee mechanics (*Magee's opedic Physical Assessment*).

ture: Note any postural abnormalities, as genu varum (bow-legged), genu um (knock-kneed), or genu recurvatum erextension of the knee). These can ate chronic issues or predispositions to ain injuries (*Orthopaedic Physical*

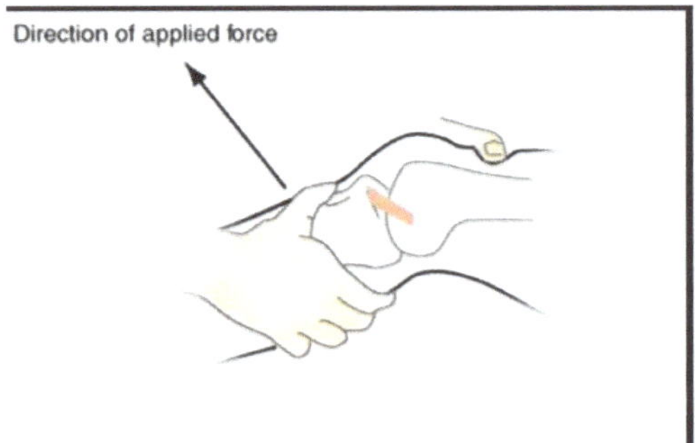

The Lachman test is conducted at 30° flexion

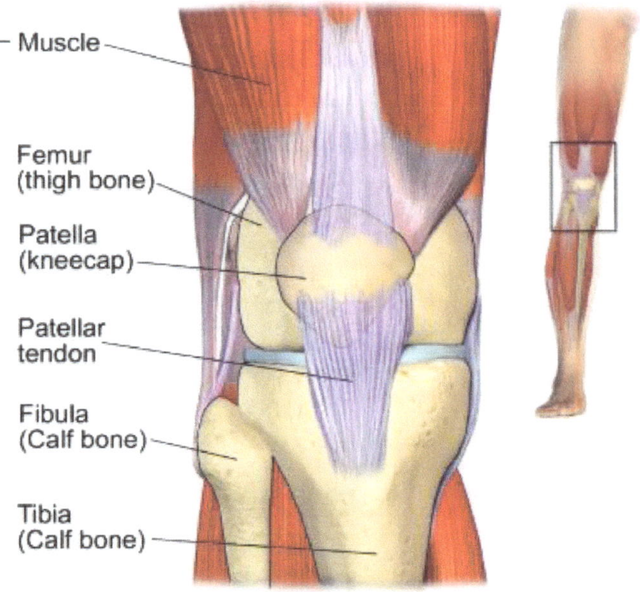

Kneecap

Local Inspection

Skin: Examine the skin for any signs of redness (erythema), swelling, bruising (ecchymosis), scars from previous surgeries or injuries, rashes, or trophic changes. Redness and warmth can Assessment). suggest inflammation or infection (*Textbook of Physical Diagnosis: History and Examination*).

Swelling: Differentiate between generalized joint effusion (fluid within the joint capsule) and localized swelling.
Effusion often presents as a ballooning of the suprapatellar pouch and obliteration of the normal contours around the patella.
Localized swelling might indicate bursitis (e.g., prepatellar or infrapatellar bursitis) or a cyst (e.g., Baker's cyst in the popliteal fossa) (*Clinical Sports Medicine*).

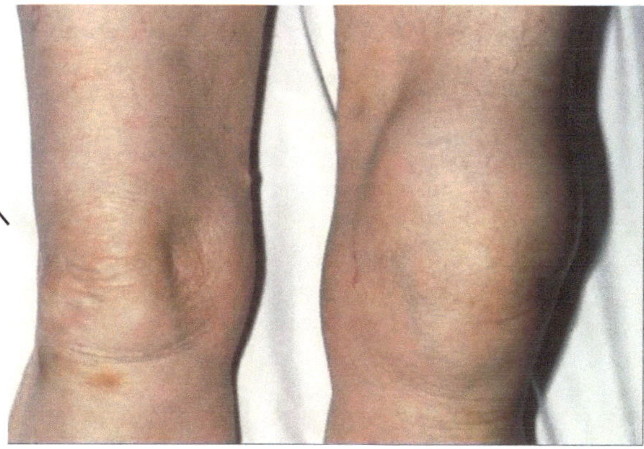

Ballottement of the Patella: This test is used to detect large effusions. With the knee extended, compress the suprapatellar pouch with one hand and then push the patella sharply against the femur with the other hand. A "floating" or "bouncing" sensation indicates significant fluid (*Clinical Examination: A Systematic Guide to Physical Diagnosis*).

Bulge Sign (or Stroke Test): For smaller effusions, milk fluid from the medial side of the patella upwards, then stroke down the lateral side. The appearance of a bulge on the medial side indicates fluid (*Magee's Orthopedic Physical Assessment*).

Medial Femoral Condyle: Palpate for tenderness.

•*Assessment*).

Medial Tibial Plateau: Palpate for tenderness.

Medial Joint Line: Palpate along the joint line for tenderness, which is a key indicator of meniscal pathology (medial meniscus tear) or medial collateral ligament (MCL) injury (*Clinical Examination: A Systematic Guide to Physical Diagnosis*).

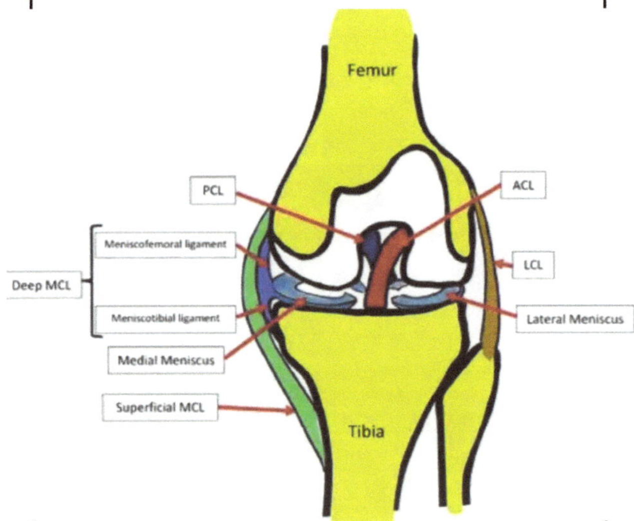

Medial Collateral Ligament (MCL): Palpate the MCL from its origin on the medial femoral epicondyle to its insertion on the medial tibia. Tenderness along its course suggests a sprain or tear (*Magee's Orthopedic Physical Assessment*).

Pes Anserine Bursa: Located on the medial aspect of the tibia, approximately 2-3 cm below the joint line. Tenderness here indicates pes anserine bursitis (*Orthopaedic Physical Assessment*).

Active Range of Motion (AROM)
Ask the patient to actively move their knee through its full range of motion.

•*Assessment*).

Flexion: Normal range is typically 0-140 degrees (*Magee's Orthopedic Physical Assessment*).

Extension: Normal range is 0 degrees (full extension), with some individuals having a few degrees of hyperextension (genu recurvatum).
Observe for any pain, stiffness, or compensatory movements during active motion.

Passive Range of Motion (PROM)
Gently move the patient's knee through its full range of motion.
Flexion: Assess the end-feel. A soft end-feel is normal due to soft tissue approximation.

Extension: Assess the end-feel. A firm end-feel is normal due to capsular and ligamentous tension.

Note any limitations in motion, pain, or crepitus. Crepitus can indicate degenerative changes or meniscal pathology (*Orthopaedic Physical Assessment*).

Goniometry: Use a goniometer to objectively measure the angles of flexion and extension, especially when tracking progress or documenting limitations (*Clinical Sports Medicine*). *Assessment*).

Passive Range of Motion (PROM)
Gently move the patient's knee through its full range of motion.
Flexion: Assess the end-feel. A soft end-feel is normal due to soft tissue approximation.

Extension: Assess the end-feel. A firm end-feel is normal due to capsular and ligamentous tension.

Assess the strength and pain response of the major muscle groups around the knee. The patient attempts to move against resistance provided by the examiner.

Knee Flexion (Hamstrings): Patient attempts to flex the knee against resistance.

Knee Extension (Quadriceps): Patient attempts to extend the knee against resistance. *Assessment*).

Pain during resisted isometric contraction without pain on passive stretch of the same muscle group can indicate tendinopathy (*Textbook of Physical Diagnosis: History and Examination*).

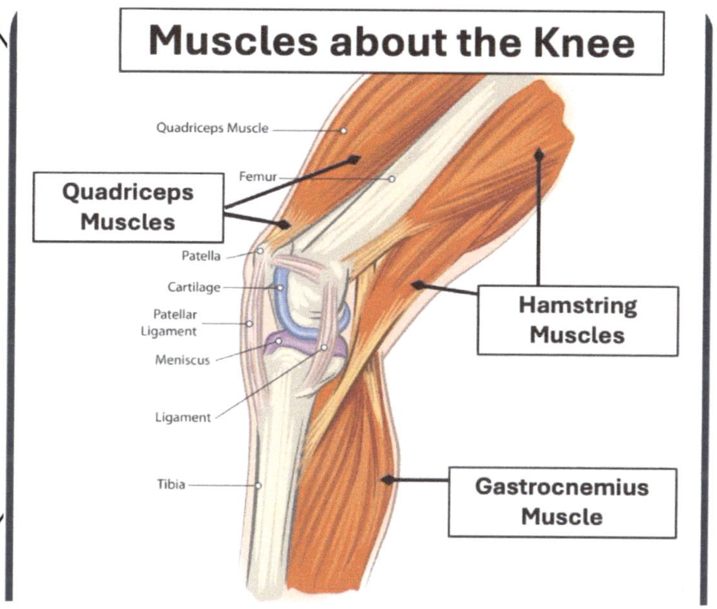

Passive Range of Motion (PROM)

Gently move the patient's knee through its full range of motion.

Flexion: Assess the end-feel. A soft end-feel is normal due to soft tissue approximation.

Extension: Assess the end-feel. A firm end-feel is normal due to capsular and ligamentous tension.

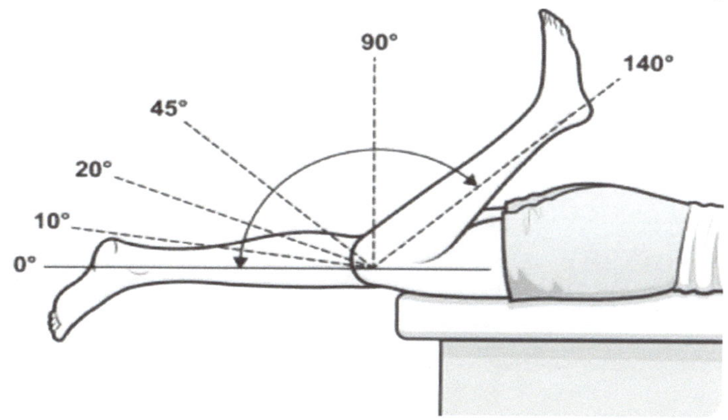

Anterior Drawer Test (ACL): With the patient supine, knee flexed to 90 degrees, and foot flat on the table, the examiner sits on the patient's foot to stabilize it. The examiner then grasps the tibia just below the joint line and pulls it anteriorly. Excessive anterior translation of the tibia indicates an ACL tear

Posterior Drawer Test (PCL): Similar position to the anterior drawer test, but the examiner pushes the tibia posteriorly. Excessive posterior translation indicates a PCL tear (*Textbook of Physical Diagnosis: History and Examination*).

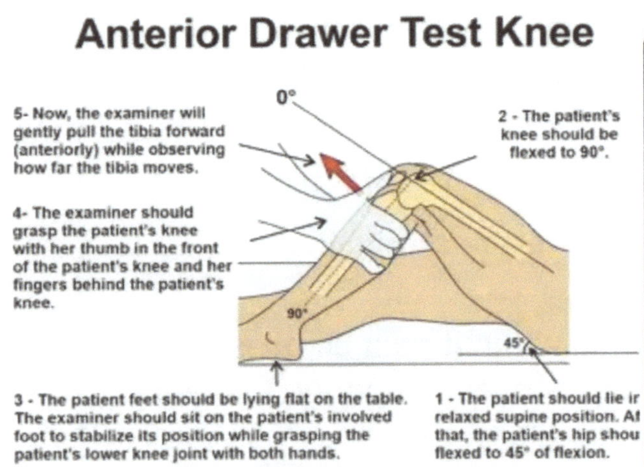

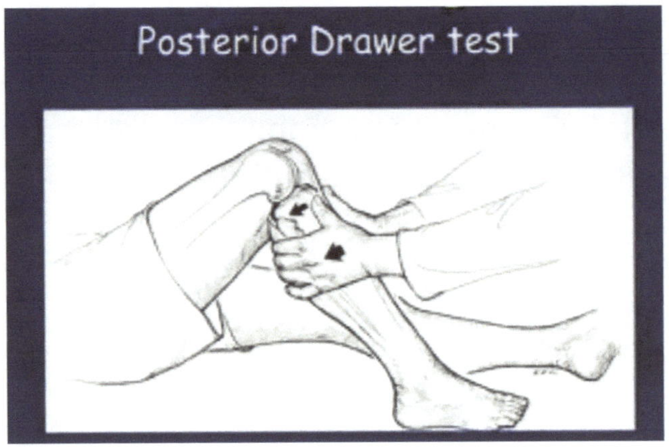

Lachman Test (ACL): This is often considered the most sensitive test for ACL integrity. With the patient supine, the knee is flexed to 20-30 degrees. The examiner stabilizes the distal femur with one hand and grasps the proximal tibia with the other, then pulls the tibia anteriorly. A soft or absent end-feel, or increased anterior translation compared to the contralateral side, indicates an ACL tear (*Magee's Orthopedic Physical Assessment*).

Meniscal Tests

McMurray Test: With the patient supine, the examiner fully flexes the knee.

Medial Meniscus: Externally rotate the tibia and apply a valgus stress while slowly extending the knee. A palpable or audible click, or pain, suggests a medial meniscal tear (*Orthopaedic Physical Assessment*).

Lateral Meniscus: Internally rotate the tibia and apply a varus stress while slowly extending the knee. A palpable or audible click, or pain, suggests a lateral meniscal tear (*Clinical Sports Medicine*).

Apley's Compression Test: With the patient prone and the knee flexed to 90 degrees, the examiner applies a downward compressive force through the heel while rotating the tibia internally and externally. Pain or a click suggests a meniscal tear (*Textbook of Physical Diagnosis: History and Examination*).

Apley's Distraction Test: In the same position, the examiner applies an upward distracting force while rotating the tibia. If pain is relieved, it further supports a meniscal injury, as distraction reduces pressure on the meniscus (*Magee's Orthopedic Physical Assessment*).

Figure 2. Examination Maneuvers

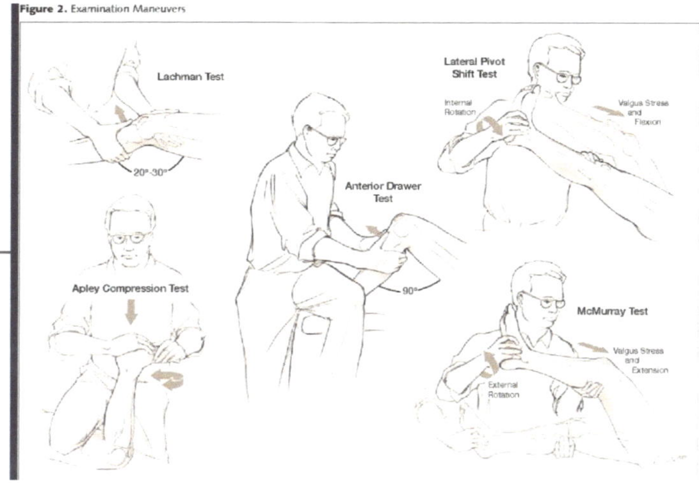

Patellar Apprehension Test: With the patient supine and the knee extended, the examiner attempts to displace the patella laterally. If the patient expresses apprehension or attempts to stop the movement, it suggests patellar instability or a history of dislocation (*Clinical Examination: A Systematic Guide to Physical Diagnosis*).

Clarke's Sign (Patellar Grind Test): With the patient supine and the knee extended, the examiner presses down on the superior pole of the patella and asks the patient to contract their quadriceps. Pain or crepitus suggests patellofemoral pain syndrome (*Orthopaedic Physical Assessment*).

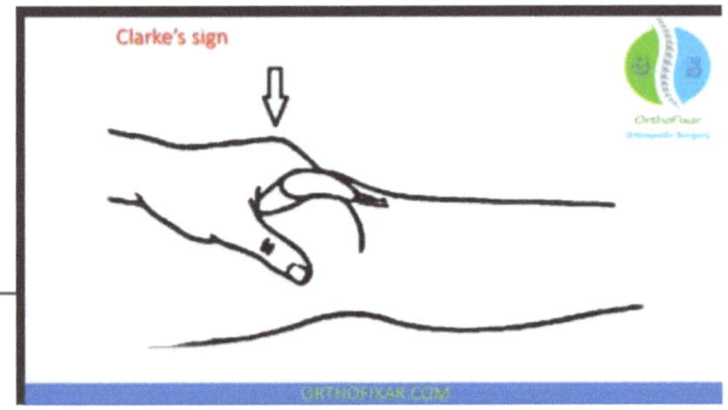

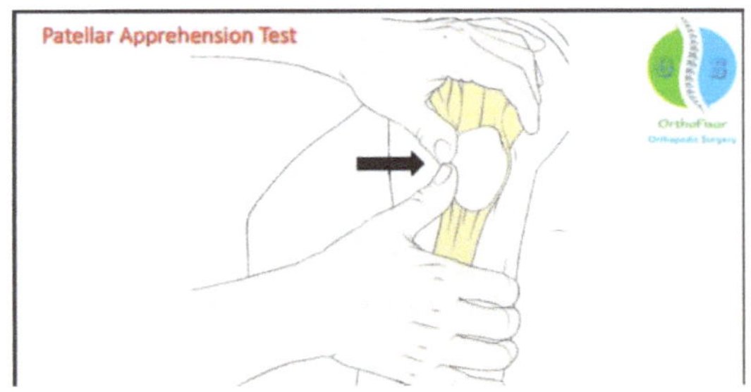

Other Special Tests

Noble Compression Test (ITB Friction Syndrome): With the patient supine, the hip and knee are flexed to 90 degrees. The examiner applies pressure over the lateral femoral epicondyle (where the ITB crosses) and slowly extends the knee. Pain at approximately 30 degrees of flexion suggests ITB friction syndrome (*Clinical Sports Medicine*).

References:

- Reference: Visual Fields – Colorado Neuroscience
- Likely Source: Anatomy teaching resources
- Likely Source: Neuro-ophthalmology education
- Commonly found in: *OphthoBook*, *EyeRounds.org*
- Commonly found in: *EyeWiki*, *Moran CORE*
- Likely Source: Eyelid pathology teaching sets
- Commonly found in: *Moran CORE*, *Kanski's Clinical Ophthalmology*
- Likely Source: Retinal pathology atlases
- Commonly found in: *EyeWiki*, *Retina Image Bank*, *Kanski's Clinical Ophthalmology*

References:

WebMD – Pictures of Swollen Feet and Ankles

Macleod's clinical examination 12th edition

Getty Images – Oxygen Cannula Stock Photos

Heart Valve Surgery – Open Heart Surgery Scars

Radiopaedia – Pectus Excavatum

Radiopaedia – open pnuemothorax

Radiopaedia – Pneumothorax

Respiratory Therapy Zone – Rhonchi Overview

Practical Clinical Skills – Egophony

- MHMedical – Thorax & Lungs Advanced Techniques

References

Stanford Medicine 25 explanation of spasticity vs rigidity. General comparison articles such as *This vs That* also cover similar diagrams

ScienceFacts – Reflex Arc overview with diagrams. Wikipedia – Reflex Arc (includes labeled diagrams similar to yours)

Physiopedia – Motor Neurone page (covers UMN/LMN features)

Physiopedia – Romberg Test page (commonly includes similar clinical illustrations)

Nursing Physical Assessment textbook (Pressbooks) – Reflex Testing section

Bullet Psych – MSE in Depression

HumanBodyPartsAnatomy.com – Brain lobes guide

HumanBodyPartsAnatomy.com – Knee Anatomy guide

TeachMeAnatomy – Knee Joint page

KneeGuru – Lachman Test page (includes hand-position diagrams)

WikiSM – Lachman's Test (includes illustrations)

Shutterstock – Swollen knee stock images

Getty Images – Swollen knee photos

NursingNotes. *Nursing Notes PDF – Nursing Study Materials.* NursingNotes.com..

Stanford Medicine 25. *Spasticity versus Rigidity: Stanford 25 Skills Symposium*. Stanford Medicine

ScienceFacts. *Reflex Arc – Definition, Steps, Components, and Diagram*. ScienceFacts.net

Upper vs Lower Motor Neuron Spectrum

Kenhub. *Motor neuron: Anatomy and structure*. Kenhub.com

Physiopedia. *Romberg Test*. Physio-pedia.com

Nursing Physical Assessment. *Reflex Testing*. Pressbooks

Human Body Parts Anatomy. *Lobes of the Brain: Complete Guide with Functions & Diagram*. humanbodypartsanatomy.com

Human Body Parts Anatomy. *Knee Anatomy: Complete Guide to Parts, Names & Diagram*. humanbodypartsanatomy.com

KneeGuru. *Lachman Test*. kneeguru.co.uk

Shutterstock. *Swollen Knee Royalty-Free Images*. shutterstock.com

OrthoFixar. *Anterior Drawer Test of the Knee*. orthofixar.com

Physiopedia. *Posterior Drawer Test (Knee)*. physio-pedia.com

Orthobullets. *Knee Physical Exam – Adult*. orthobullets.com

OrthoFixar. *Patellar Grind Test (Clarke Sign)*. orthofixar.com

Clinical Spectrum of Upper and Lower Motor Neuron Involvement – Unlabeled (Image ID: 79876). Available at: https://www.netterimages.com/clinical-spectrum-of-upper-and-lower-motor-neuron-involvement-unlabeled-79876.html

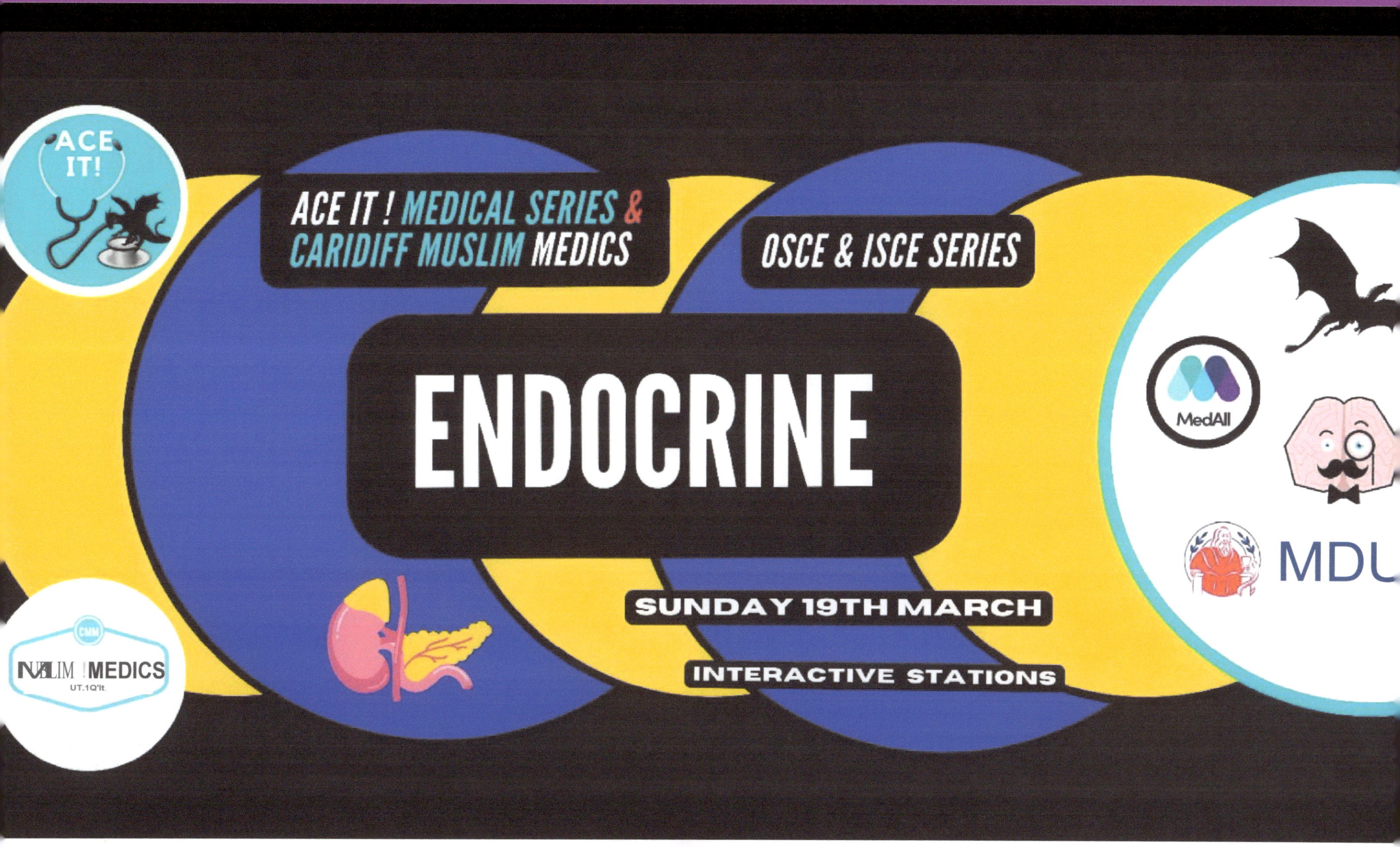
ACE IT!
ACE IT ! MEDICAL SERIES &
CARIDIFF MUSLIM MEDICS
OSCE & ISCE SERIES
ENDOCRINE
SUNDAY 19TH MARCH
INTERACTIVE STATIONS
MedAll
MDU

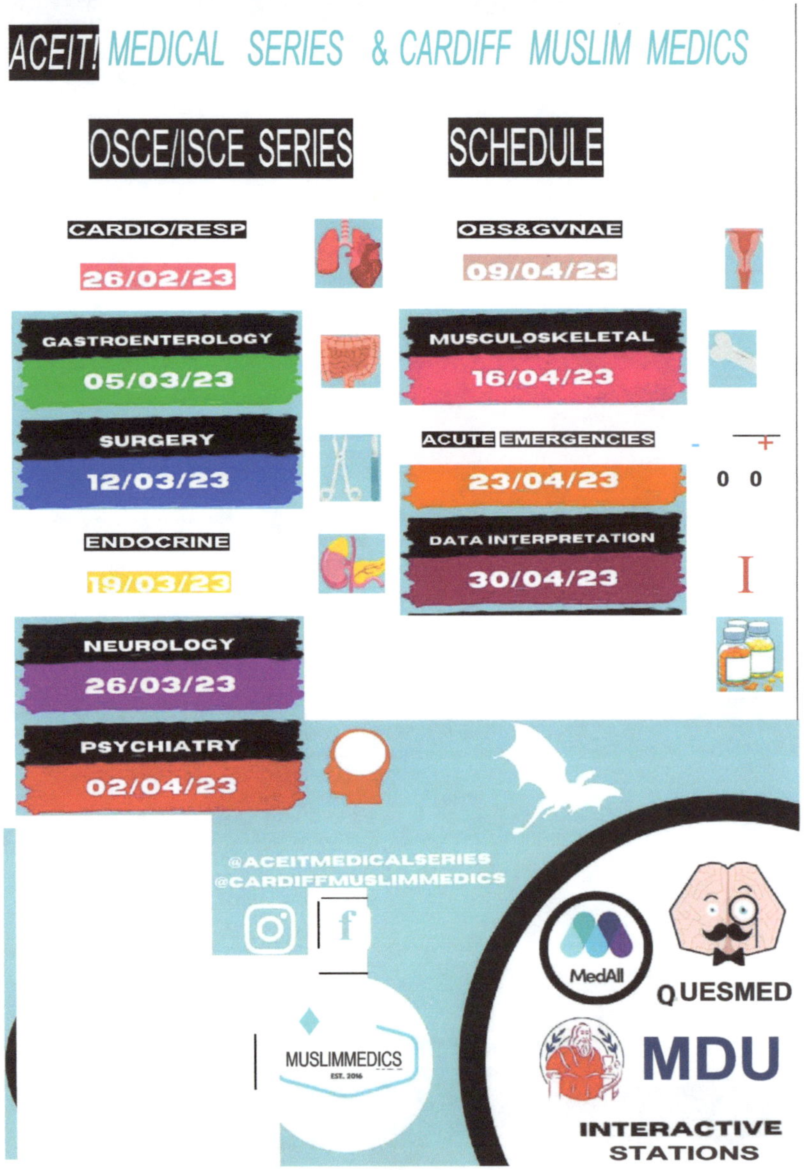
ACEIT! MEDICAL SERIES & CARDIFF MUSLIM MEDICS
OSCE/ISCE SERIES SCHEDULE
CARDIO/RESP
26/02/23
GASTROENTEROLOGY
05/03/23
SURGERY
12/03/23
ENDOCRINE
19/03/23
NEUROLOGY
26/03/23
PSYCHIATRY
02/04/23
OBS&GVNAE
09/04/23
MUSCULOSKELETAL
16/04/23
ACUTE EMERGENCIES
23/04/23
DATA INTERPRETATION
30/04/23
@ACEITMEDICALSERIES
@CARDIFFMUSLIMMEDICS
MUSLIMMEDICS
EST. 2016
MedAll
QUESMED
MDU
INTERACTIVE STATIONS

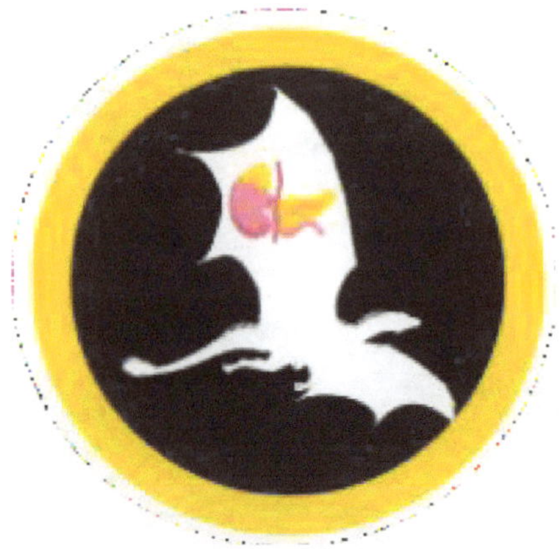

Learning Outcomes

Confidence in Passing your OSCEs

History Taking

PC

HPC

PMH

FH

DH – ALLERGIES

SH – smoking, ADLs, illicit substances ICE

Paeds – Birth, Feeding, Growth, Development, Immunisations, Social Services Psych – Suicide risk?, Risk to others?

O+G – Foetal movements felt, Rhesus Status Systemic enquiry and Red Flags

You should know how to perform a thyroid exam

3	echn·cal performance	rong mask selected. Did not aspirate _rio .·njecting Wrong nee . le use. Wrong dosage of medication injec ed. **Did not c ec , ame on char** Not cleaning finger wit wa er p ior checking blood glucose Faj u e to correctly d·spose of sharps.

Station 1

Student Briefing	You are a 4th year medical student working in A&E
Setting	A&E Department
Patient Details	This 14 year old female patient presents with a history of abdominal pain
Task	Please take a brief history from the patient. You will then be asked some questions and asked to perform a clinical skill.

History

S: All over tummy
O: Morning 8am when I woke up
C: Sharp pains
R: Nil
A: Vomiting, vomited 3 times this morning
T: 8am
E/R: Paracetamol, vomited it up
S: 8/10
PC Abdo pain and vomiting
HPC Fever in last wk, tired. Sporadic onset. Some shortness of breath associated.
PMH Nil. **SH** Smokes with friends
DH Nil. No allergies **FH** Nil
LMP 14d ago, cycles regular.
Safeguarding

On examination the patient has generalised abdominal pain and dehydrated with dry mucous membranes, pyrexial.

Here is the NEWS chart.

Based on your history, clinical findings and chart, what would be your list of differential diagnoses at this stage?
How would you investigate?

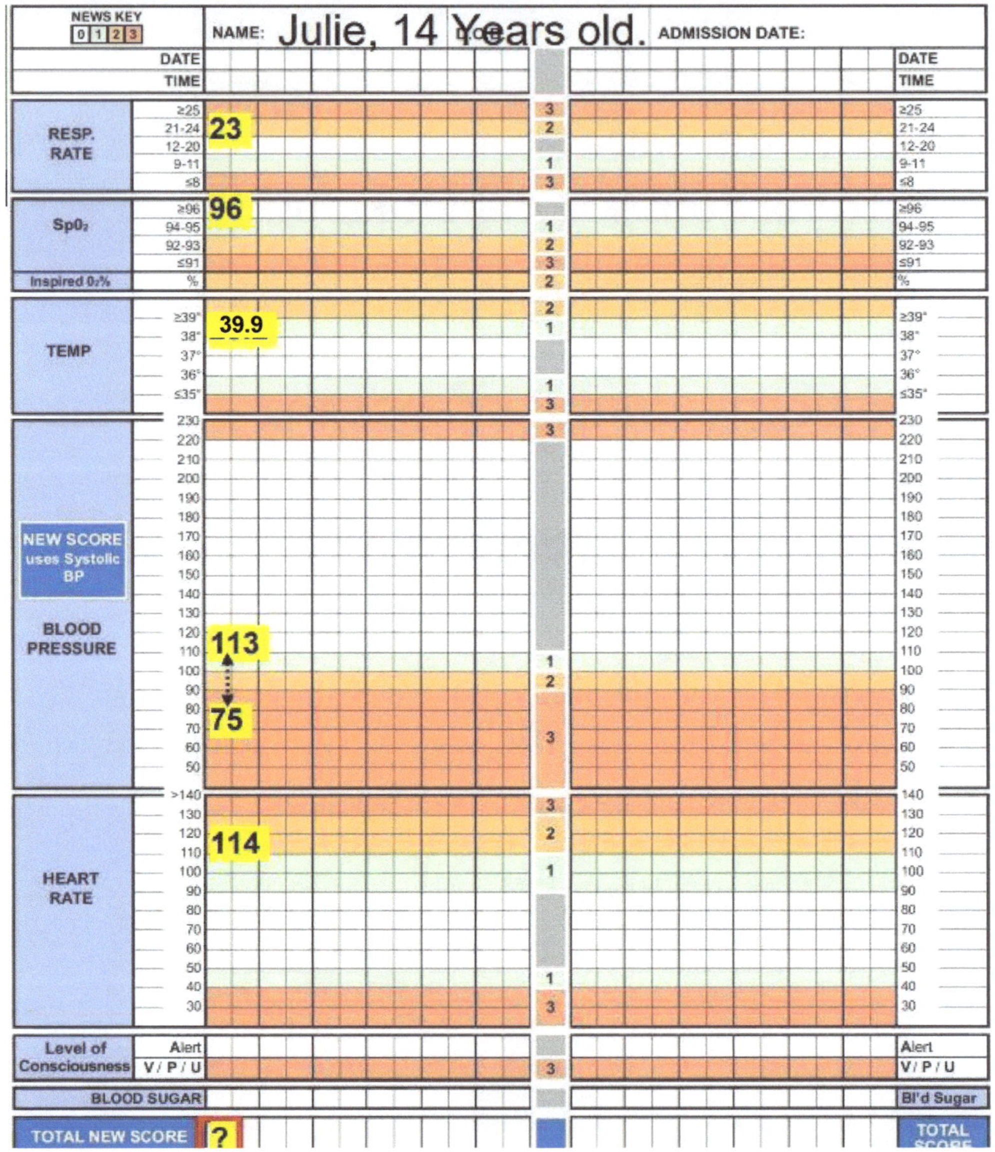

Investigations

Bedside:

History, examination, A-E assessment, NEWS chart, ECG, Urinalysis, MC&S, Pregnancy test

Bloods:

FBC, U&E, CRP, ABG/VBG (lactate), blood ketones, blood culture

Imaging

CXR (chest infection), Abdominal USS (gynae)

PREGNANCY TEST

Julie Adams

DOB: 12/03/2009

Taken 12/03/2023

Urinalysis:

pH 6.5

Leukocytes ++

Nitrite +

Ketones ++

Protein 0

Glucose +++

Arterial Blood Gas:

pH 7.26 (7.35-7.45)

PaO2 11.2 (11-13)

PaCO2 4.2 (4.7-6)

HCO3 19 (24-30)

BE -4 (-2 to +2)

Blood Glucose 16 (4-11.1)

Pregnancy test Negative

Management

Diabetic Ketoacidosis – **Acute management**

Manage patient in A-E approach, call for help and escalate to senior and medical on call, following local DKA protocol.

1. Fluid replacement
2. Insulin - Fixed rate insulin infusion 0.1kg/hr

Correct electrolytes. K^+ replacement. Glucose.

Start sub cut insulin 1hr before stopping fixed rate insulin infusion

Medical – Insulin regime

Conservative – Educate and safety net. Hypoglycaemia – insulin induced. Sick day rules. Educate on uncontrolled sugar levels. MDT approach. Informing school, dietician, diabetic nurse. ?social. DAFNE course type 1 diabetes.

Surgical - NA

Station 2

Student Briefing	You are a 4th year medical student working in A&E
Setting	Antenatal Clinic
Patient Details	This 28 year old Mum to be presents for a visit
Task	Please take a brief history from the patient. You will then be asked some questions and asked to perform a clinical skill.

History

Aysha Azaan. 03/03/1993.

PC – Presenting for a check up in antenatal dept. 34week.

G1P1 – going fine

Foetal movements felt. Rh +ve.

HOPC – kid are looking forward to new sibling at home

PMH – HTN

FH – Diabetes in Mum. No pre eclampsia

DH – Folic acid 500 mg. Labetalol. Aspirin

SH – Fine

Babies. Cervical Smear. Menstrual periods. Scans fine. Previous pregnancy born at terms no issues.

Investigations

Bedside: History, Routine Obstetrics exam. CTG.

Bloods: OGTT at 24-28 weeks in women with risk factors, random blood glucose, HbA1C (Completed after diagnosis of diagnosis of GDM to identify women with overt T2DM)

Imaging: Foetal US

Aysha Azaan
03/03/1993
Gestational Chart

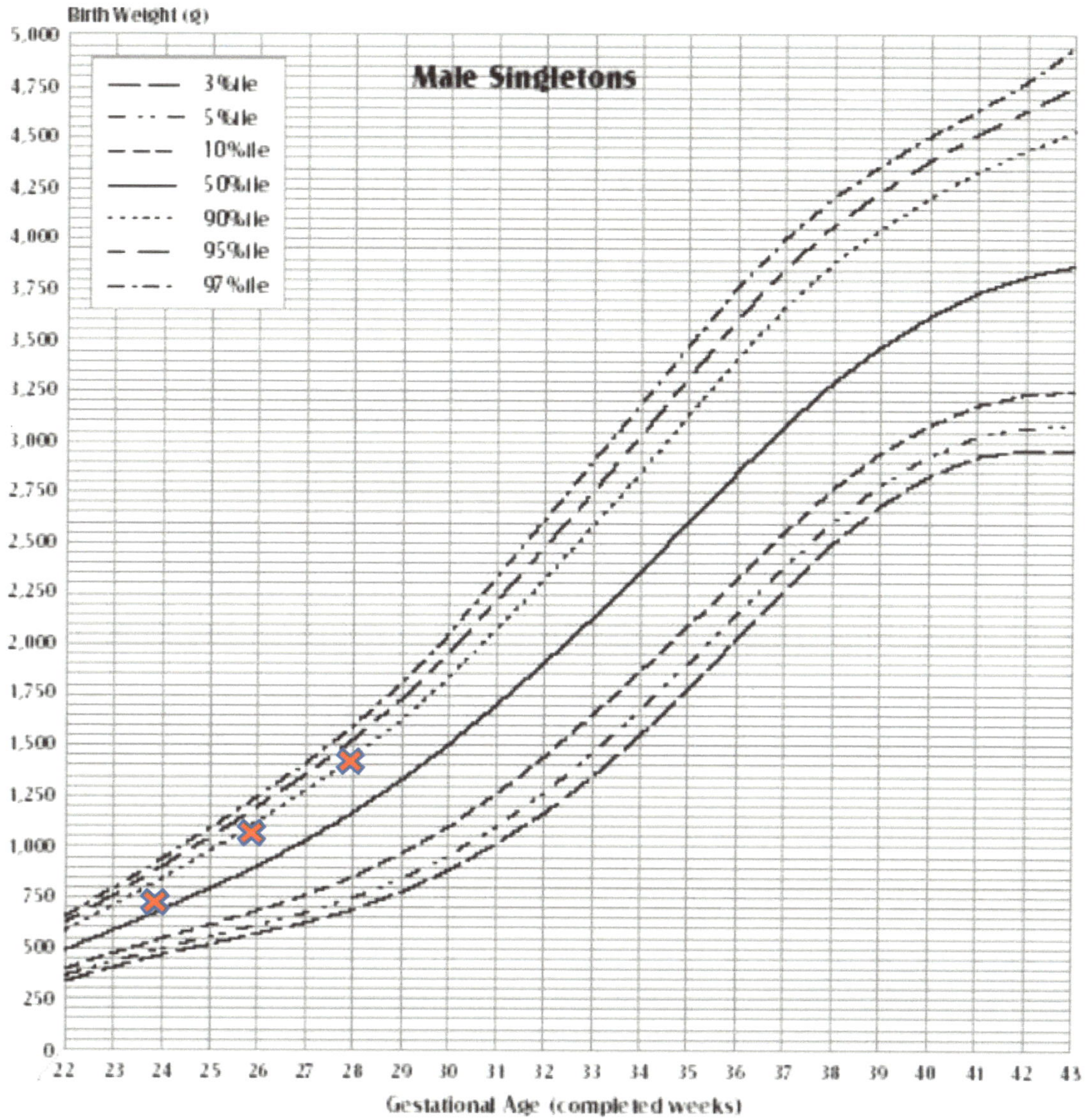

Management

Medical – Depending on fasting plasma glucose, can include a combination of metformin, insulin and diet/exercise.

Surgical – US more regularly completed for foetal growth and amniotic fluid (used in planning route of delivery – C-section/Vaginal delivery)

Conservative - Refer to O+G – for consultant led follow up and review, advice and counselling regarding condition and importance in monitoring foetal movements

Station 3

Student Briefing	You are a 4th year medical student working in General Practice
Sting	General Practice
Patient Details	38 year old female with generalise tiredness over past 2 months
Task	Please take a brief history from the patient. You will then be asked some questions and asked to perform a clinical skill.

History

PC - A 40-year-old female presents with generalised tiredness over the past 2 months

HOPC - Tiredness always for the past 2 months, feel like "I don't have the energy I once did and I can't do anything". Tearful about situation as you had to stop working.

Mention you are in bed a lot as you are tired - but you are in bed, because you feel cold and need to wear extra layers to keep warm.

Weight gain of 4-5 kg over the past 2 months - no change in eating.

If asked - have experienced heavy periods in the past 2 months.

Feels constipated at times, but it is not a major issue.

No loss of blood anywhere, no fever, no previous issues similar to this, no fever or night sweats, no recent viral illness, no goitre present on exam, no trauma

Ensure they take risk history: No suicidal ideation, No history of self harm, No psychotic or delusional symptoms.

PMH - T1D, RA

FH - Sister has Coeliac

DH - Nill, allergy to penicillin causes rash on hands

SH - Smokes 5 cigarettes a day for 10 years, tried to stop unsuccessful

Investigations

Bedside:

History, Basic observations, ECG, Urinalysis, Pregnancy test

Bloods:

FBC, U&E, CRP, TFTs, anti-TPO, U&Es, Mental risk assessment, tumour markers

Imaging:

Thyroid US, Radioiodine scan (specialist)

Differential Diagnoses

TFT's

Rasheeda Qureshi DOB: 12/03/1983
Taken: 12/03/2023

TSH	15.1 mU/l
T3 T4	2.1 8
Anti-TSH receptor stimulating antibodies	Negative
Anti-thyroid peroxidase antibodies	Positive

TSH: 0.4-4.0 mU/L[2]
Free T4: 9 - 24 pmol/L
Free T3: 3.5 - 7.8 pmol/L

Management

How would you manage this patient?

Conservative – Education and counselling of condition and treatment, Risk assessment, Refer to Endocrine team, Consider occupational therapy – regarding her work. Blood tests.

Medical – Levothyroxine

Surgical – Not indicated in managing primary hypothyroidism

Station 4

Student Briefing	You are a 4th year medical student working in A&E
Setting	A&E Department
Patient Details	30 year old male presents with recent confusion
Task	Please take a brief history from the patient. You will then be asked some questions and asked to perform a clinical skill.

History

PC - 60 year old male Mohammed presents with recent confusion, take a collateral history from his wife

HOPC: Is confused, so talking to his wife. Hasn't been able to talk and have a conversation with her for 2 days - doesn't know where he is. Confused for 2 days.

Mentions for the past 4 days has had a temperature - complained of abdominal discomfort and vomiting (no blood, bile in vomit) "many times" over last 2 days.

Bowels are loose for the past 2 days - no blood, not black in colour.

'Only when asked about skin changes' - "I have noticed the skin on palm of his hands have started to darken"

Has not been able to eat or drink, no trauma, no weight loss, no visual or joint changes, no urinary dysfunction, no bowel dysfunction

PMH: Nill

FH: Nill

DH: Nill, no allergies

SH: smokes 10/day for 40 years.

Investigations

Interpret these results below:

Temp: 39, RR: 23, BP: 85/60, HR - 120 , O2 - 91%, WBC - 12.3 (4.00 - 11.00)

Na+	124 mmol/l	(135 - 145)
K+	6.6 mmol/l	(3.5 - 5.0)
Bicarbonate	26 mmol/L	(22 - 29)
Urea	4.3 mmol/L	(2.0 - 7.0)
Creatinine	105 µmol/L	(55 - 120)
Calcium	2.4 mmol/L	(2.1 - 2.6)
Fasting glucose	5.3 mmol/L	(4 - 7)

Mohammed Kamal 02/01/1963
Test Taken: 12/03/2023

SBAR

Complete an SBAR for this Addisonian Crisis secondary to Sepsis (most likely from abdominal infection)

Management

Conservative: Call for senior support, refer to appropriate team

Medical: A-E, Sepsis 6 protocol – antibiotics according to local health board guidelines, adrenal insufficiency management (hydrocortisone 100 mg IM or IV - continue hydrocortisone 6 hourly until the patient is stable), consider fludrocortisone.

Surgical: May be necessary depending on the underlying cause of the abdominal infection

Long term – steroid replacements required (hydrocortisone and fludrocortisone), counselling and education on condition and treatment. Safety bracelet. Educating on sick days

Thank You

www.ingramcontent.com/pod-product-compliance
Lightning Source LLC
LaVergne TN
LVHW070818210926
848482LV00004B/286